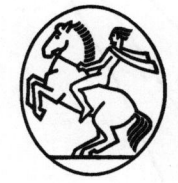

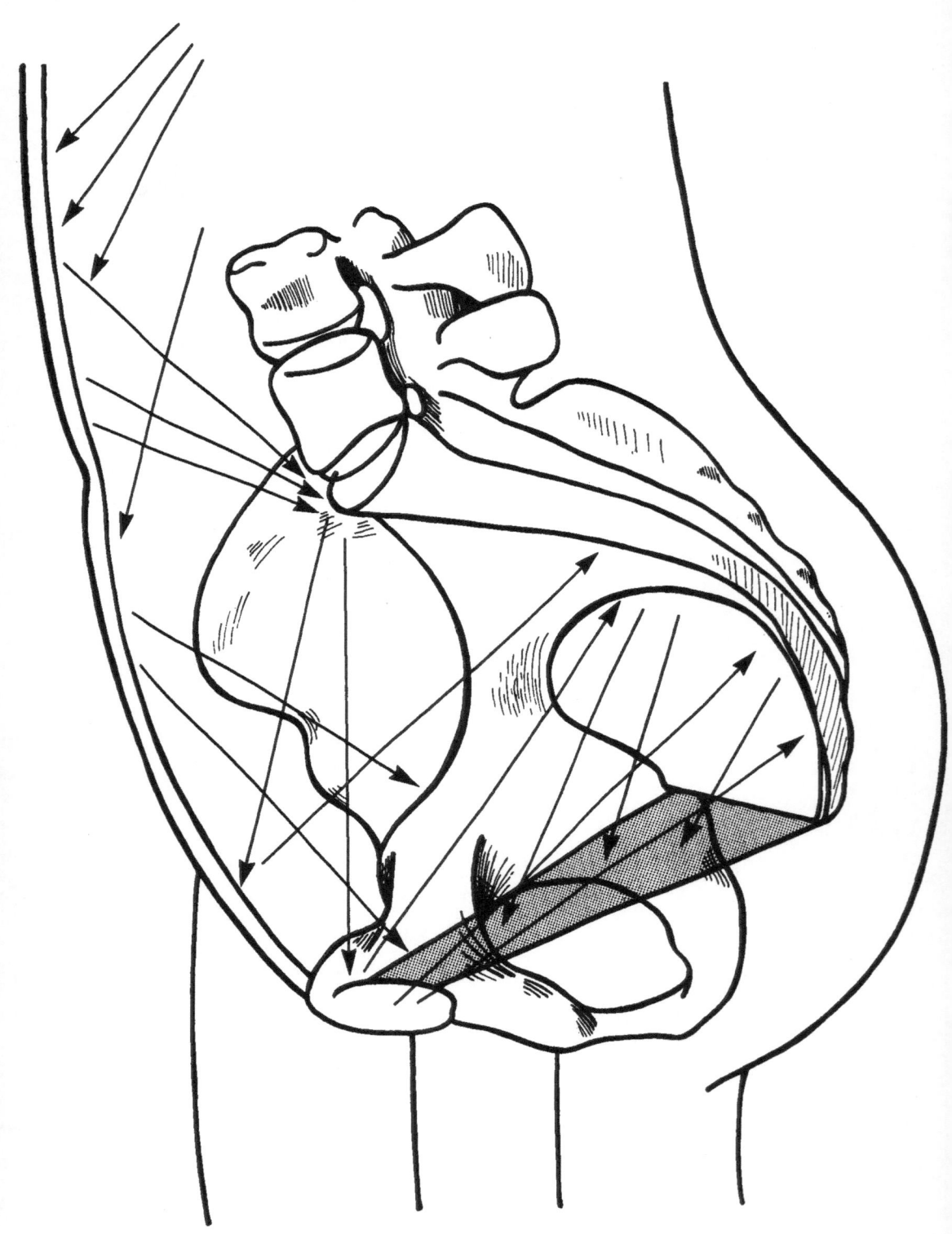

Robert F. Zacharin

Pelvic Floor Anatomy and the Surgery of Pulsion Enterocoele

With a Foreword by
Richard E. Symmonds
Mayo Clinic

Springer-Verlag Wien GmbH

Robert F. Zacharin,
M.G.O. (Melb.), F.R.C.S. (Eng.), F.R.C.O.G., F.R.A.C.S., F.R.A.C.O.G.
Gynecologist in Charge, Department of Gynecology, Alfred Hospital, Melbourne, Australia

© 1985 by Springer-Verlag Wien
Originally published by Springer- Verlag Wien New York in 1985
Softcover reprint of the hardcover 1st edition 1985

With 75 partly coloured Figures

Cover design: Joachim Böning, Vienna, Austria
Frontispiece: Routes of dispersion of intraabdominal pressure in the erect human. The key role of the lumbo-sacral joint is emphasized, and also that of the bony pelvis and sacrum. Levator ani is indicated by the darkened triangular area in the pelvic floor.

Library of Congress Cataloging in Publication Data: Zacharin, Robert Fyfe. Pelvic floor anatomy and the surgery of pulsion enterocoele. 1. Uterus—Prolapse—Surgery. 2. Generative organs, Female—Anatomy. 3. Gynecology, Operative. I. Title. [DNLM: 1. Genitalia, Female—anatomy & histology. 2. Hernia—surgery. 3. Uterine Prolapse—surgery. 3. Uterine Prolapse—surgery. WP 250 Z16p] RG361.Z33 1985. 618.1'44. 85-17268

ISBN 978-3-7091-4077-2   ISBN 978-3-7091-4075-8 (eBook)
DOI 10.1007/978-3-7091-4075-8

To Tricia

"Have you guessed the riddle yet?" the Hatter said, turning to Alice again.
"No, I give it up," Alice replied: "what's the answer?"
"I haven't the slightest idea," said the Hatter.
"Nor I," said the Hare.
Alice sighed wearily. "I think you might do something better with the time," she said, "than waste it asking riddles with no answers."

Alice's Adventures in Wonderland, Lewis Carroll, 1865

Foreword

It is in the surgical aspect of their specialty that the gynecologists' work may be most frequently judged by their peers or by the litigious society that currently exists. Great and commendable progress has been made over the past 30 years in the basic scientific, endocrinologic and obstetric aspects of the specialty, but this has occurred with a commensurate de-emphasis of surgical procedures and surgical training, a decline in devotion to technical detail and perfection, and a tendency to take surgery for granted.

Obstetric and gynecologic residency programs provide increasing numbers of specialists with average competence in the performance of the common, rather standardized gynecologic operations. In general, technical skill in the extirpative operations can be acquired far more readily than proficiency in the art of reconstructive surgery.

At present, for a number of reasons, gynecologic surgical training is most deficient in regard to the surgical correction of severe forms of obstetrically damaged genital tract supports. The operations for prolapse defy standardization and require great technical individualization; this must be based on the surgeon's judgment developed through experience, a thorough understanding of normal pelvic anatomy, and recognition of the deficiency responsible for the prolapse in individual cases.

Unfortunately, mere technical competence in the accomplishment of abdominal and vaginal hysterectomy does not ensure the recognition of these deficiencies; when they are recognized, the surgical correction of them may be inadequate. More than 700,000 hysterectomies are accomplished in the United States each year. It has been estimated that 1 per 250 to 300 of these patients subsequently will have some degree of vaginal vault prolapse and enterocoele. In my experience and that of others, the number of patients referred with recurrent prolapse has been increasing each year, which serves to emphasize the importance of this new book, Pelvic Floor Anatomy and the Surgery of Pulsion Enterocoele. To my knowledge, thisrepresents the first volume devoted exclusively to this topic.

Over a period of many years, the author of this book, a man of experience, insight, and recognized surgical talents, has reported detailed studies of comparative pelvic anatomy in the female. An understanding of this anatomy is of the utmost importance in any consideration of the etiologic and therapeutic aspects of prolapse, enterocoele, urinary incontinence, and other gynecologic conditions that require reconstructive efforts. Included in the monograph is an informative and remarkably complete historic review of the diverse operative procedures, largely empirically developed, that have been devised for the correction of prolapse.

Careful study and thoughtful consideration of the anatomic concepts proposed and the operative techniques suggested and beautifully illustrated in this unique volume will be invaluable not only for the resident physician but also for the specialist-practitioner who performs "routine" operations for prolapse but may infrequently encounter or not feel qualified to perform the complex operative procedures required for the correction of the unusual, massive and recurrent forms of pelvic herniations.

Richard E. Symmonds, M. D.
Emeritus Chairman,
Division of Gynecologic Surgery,
Mayo Clinic and Mayo Foundation;
Emeritus Professor of Gynecologic Surgery,
Mayo Medical School,
Rochester, Minnesota,
U. S. A.

Preface

Pulsion enterocoele is a most distressing and serious complication of pelvic surgery and may follow vaginal hysterectomy, abdominal hysterectomy or the Manchester operation. It appears to be most common after vaginal hysterectomy and certainly this procedure is associated with the largest examples of the problem, despite many surgical precautions advocated to prevent its appearance. It has become clear that poor quality genital tract supports are to blame rather than the surgeon.

Once a large vaginal inversion has developed it cannot be managed conservatively, for the inherent risk of rupture is great, since the peritoneal cavity and outside world are separated only by vaginal wall and the peritoneum. A multitude of measures to correct the situation by surgery have been advocated over many years, so clearly no one technique has emerged which can supply all the answers.

Management depends on several important considerations which include, the age of the patient and her ability to tolerate surgery and whether or not vaginal function is to be preserved. Available surgical techniques include the vaginal approach, an abdominal approach or a combination, and just what procedure a gynecologist chooses depends upon his belief regarding the supportive anatomy of the genital tract and accordingly either an entirely empirical or attempted specific attack will be made.

In many facets of surgical therapy in different parts of the body, for reasons difficult to discern, an empirical approach unrelated to the anatomy concerned is most popular and this has certainly been the case with pulsion enterocoele. Convinced that the correct approach to the surgical correction of large pulsion enterocoele must lie in a specific attempt to reconstruct the normal supporting anatomy of the upper genital tract, abdominoperineal correction was commenced in 1968.

The publications of Berglas and Rubin on levator myography indicated with clarity just how the levator complex and pelvic cellular tissue support functioned, and was the basis upon which the procedure was designed. There has been a great deal of controversy about genital tract supports since the turn of the century but gradually the situation has cleared and presently a combined role for the pelvic cellular tissues and levator complex is accepted.

This monograph discusses the anatomy of the pelvic floor in detail beginning with its evolutionary development, through normal, comparative and functional anatomy since such a view is necessary to appreciate fully the vital functional roles of the two components of upper genital tract support. Following the clinical picture of pulsion enterocoele the various methods of correction which have been proposed are examined, and finally a detailed explanation of abdominoperineal repair is given.

Large pulsion enterocoele supposedly is a rare condition, yet since 1968, 122 women have been accepted for surgical correction. If vaginal function is no longer required, total colpocleisis is the least traumatic procedure which will control the situation, and in this series was performed 25 times. A majority of the patients wished to retain vaginal function and the longterm results of abdominoperineal repair are presented in 97 women, showing clearly the excellent functional result attainable. Major surgery is required for any major surgical problem and of course there will be attendant risks and complications; but in this series they have been few. Whilst most patients come from Melbourne, a significant number have been referred from many parts of Australia, as the benefits of the technique have become known.

I am indebted to my colleague Nicholas Hamilton for his ready help and advice and particularly his surgical skill as my abdominal collaborator, to the Audiovisual Department at the Alfred Hospital (Cam Harvey, Michael Cardamone, and Angela Leaman) for the excellent photographic prints and line drawings, to Enid Meldrum, Chief Librarian in the Medical Library at the Alfred Hospital, for her expert help with references and the bibliography, to both Norman Beischer and Robert Marshall who read the initial manuscript and offered extremely helpful criticism and corrections and finally to my secretary Rosemary Stewart who has cheerfully typed the manuscript so many times.

Robert F. Zacharin
Melbourne, July 1985

Contents

Acknowledgements

(i) Figures 6 and 7: reprinted with permission of American Journal of Obstetrics & Gynecology, "Man's assumption of the erect posture." J. W. Davies. *70*, 1012 (1955).

(ii) Figures 8 and 9: by permission of Surgery, Gynecology & Obstetrics.

(iii) Figure 10: reprinted with permission of American Journal of Obstetrics & Gynecology, "Surgical significance of the recto-vaginal septum." D. H. Nicholls and P. S. Milley. *108*, 215 (1970).

(iv) Figure 11: reprinted with permission of the Annals of the Royal College of Surgeons of England.

(v) Figures 12, 13, 31: reprinted with permission of the Journal of Investigative Urology *13*, 175 (1975).

(vi) Figure 14: reprinted with permission of the Journal of Anatomy (S.F. Ayoub, The anterior fibres of levator ani in Man. Cambridge University Press.)

(vii) Figures 15, 16, 18, 20a: reprinted with permission from the American College of Obstetricians and Gynecologists. Obstetrics & Gynecology *55*, 135 (1980).

(viii) Figures 21, 22, 23, 24b, 69c, 71b, 72: reprinted with permission of the Australian and New Zealand Journal of Obstetrics and Gynaecology.

(ix) Figures 29, 30: reprinted by permission of Surgery, Gynecology & Obstetrics.

(x) Figures 32, 33: reprinted with permission from the American College of Obstetricians and Gynecologists. Obstetrics & Gynecology *15*, 711 (1960), *29*, 450 (1967).

(xi) Figures 39, 40: reprinted by permission of Annals of Surgery *133*, 255 (1951).

(xii) Figure 42: reprinted with permission from the American College of Obstetricians and Gynecologists. Obstetrics & Gynecology *32*, 802 (1968).

(xiii) Figures 53 a & b, 54, 55 a, b, c: reprinted with permission from the American College of Obstetricians and Gynecologists. Obstetrics & Gynecology *10*, 595 (1957).

(xiv) Figures 56, 57, 58, 59, 60: reprinted with permission from the American Journal of Obstetrics & Gynecology, "Vaginal prolapse following hysterectomy." R. E. Symmonds & J. E. Pratt. *79*, 899 (1960).

(xv) Figures 46, 65, 66, 68, 69 b, 75: reprinted with permission from the American College of Obstetricians and Gynecologists. Obstetrics & Gynecology *55*, 141 (1980).

Introduction

Since earliest medical records (Ebers Papyrus, 1550 B.C.) genital prolapse has been mentioned in medical literature, and for a similar period, methods of management have been described. (Emge and Durfee, 1966). Throughout the history of genital prolapse including enterocoele, the characteristic feature of writings concerned with aetiological factors, functional anatomy of genital tract supports, and methods of conservative or operative correction, has been an almost uniform empirical approach. The scientific approach came only much later and even now, the thickness of empirical overlay upon scientific knowledge, is noteworthy.

Enterocoele as an entity was mentioned first by the Frenchman R. J. C. de Garengeot in 1736, when he used the term "enterocoele vaginale". Sir Astley Cooper, the famous British anatomist surgeon, gave a classic description of the condition, as accurate today as it was then. Nomenclature of genital prolapse has been a problem since these early descriptions, the major difficulty being the wide variety of synonyms applied to the same anatomical defect. Thomas (1885) described five varieties of herniae which could present in the vagina or at the vulva — cystocoele, rectocoele, vaginal enterocoele, pudendal enterocoele and perineal enterocoele. Vaginal enterocoele meant descent of intestines into the pelvic cavity, either in front of or posterior to the broad ligament of one side, the intestines never descending directly in the median line anteriorly or posteriorly, because of the intimate vaginal relations at these points. The intestines descended always a little obliquely and more frequently posteriorly, usually the intestines alone descending in the hernial protrusion, but occasionally accompanied by omentum. Read (1951) divided enterocoele into traction and pulsion types, traction being the usual accompaniment of uterovaginal or rectal prolapse, whereas pulsion enterocoele resulted from intraabdominal pressure acting upon a congenitally deep cul-de-sac, usually in association with some inferior anatomical weakness. Some French writers have divided hernia of the labia majora or pudendal enterocoele into two varieties — anterior labial hernia or that which eventuates from the inguinal form, and posterior labial hernia or labiovaginal hernia, or hernia formed by extension of the peritoneum down in front of the broad ligament alongside the vagina to the vulva.

Kinzel (1960) defined enterocoele as any herniation of small bowel into the vagina. It was a true hernia, not a sliding hernia and as such possessed a sac, neck and contents, the neck lying between the uterosacral ligaments, anterior to the sacrum and behind the cervix. Rarely an anterior enterocoele dissected between bladder and uterus. It was his opinion that where a redundant cul-de-sac finished and an enterocoele began, was of academic interest only.

Nicholls (1969) regarded prolapse as an upper vaginal inversion, or a lower vaginal eversion. Inversion followed obstetric injury and comprised cystocoele, vault descent and traction enterocoele, but usually rectocoele was absent. Eversion followed pelvic and uro-genital diaphragm damage, and could be post-obstetric or post-menopausal in origin. Should both conditions occur in association, the vagina both inverted from above and rolled out from below.

Enterocoele known also as pouch of Douglas hernia or cul-de-sac hernia was defined by Weed and Tyrone (1950) as "a sac of peritoneum which dissected beyond its lower normal limits between the vaginal wall anteriorly and the rectum behind, to emerge through the vaginal entrance. The abdominal opening of the sac lay between the uterosacral ligaments in close proximity to the posterior aspect of the cervix." They termed it "posterior vaginal hernia". Enterocoele might be seen posterior, anterior or lateral to the vagina with or without vaginal vault inversion. It was a herniation of the peritoneal cavity, with or without portions of its contents, in areas of the pelvis where they are not normally found (Nicholls, 1972).

When aetiology was considered, most writers beginning with Thomas (1885) believed the underlying problem was parturition. All the pelvic tissues were hypertrophied greatly and relaxed during pregnancy, but with the violent efforts of child expulsion, the relaxed parts were strained.

Daniel Jones (1916) emphasized the relationship of a deep cul-de-sac to rectal and uterine prolapse. He considered a deep cul-de-sac essential for the development of vaginal enterocoele — the congenital type arose from a failure of the normal ascending obliterative process which occurred with advancing maturity and the acquired, more common type, was seen in multiparae and probably related to pregnancy.

Bueermann (1932) suggested most vaginal enterocoeles were acquired, with the trauma of childbirth as a main factor, since over 90 % of his patients had borne children. He believed congenital weakness of pelvic floor muscles and fascia could explain the rare occurrence of vaginal hernia, after such a normal physiological process as pregnancy. His theory also presupposed primary elongation of the cul-de-sac as the starting point, and he remarked further on the number of points of resemblence between the inguinal canal, and the pelvic floor and vagina. Both opened into the lower end of the abdominal cavity and both ran from the cavity almost at right angles to abdominal pressure. Both canals were covered by two main layers with a ring in each layer, and an axis which changed its obliquity, depending on the size of the mass distending the passage.

As the foetus neared term, a gradual fusion of the dorsiventral walls of the pouch of Douglas, commenced caudally (Read, 1951). The process of fusion varied in different individuals and gradations from complete nonfusion to the normal were encountered. This of course explained variability of depth of the sac. Pressure on the sac floor in an infant could re-open this fusion and furthermore it could be shown in adults that the rectovaginal septum was only this fused peritoneal process. Therefore it appeared that a congenitally deep sac frequently was present from birth, and analogy with the preformed sac of hernias became obvious.

Porges et al. (1960) considered that structures contributing to support of the pelvic organs, acted in certain respects like the components of a simple mechanical valve, and insufficiency of this valve was linked to the pathogenesis of uterine prolapse and pelvic relaxation. Nicholls (1972) believed iatrogenic alteration of pelvic anatomy could play a role also. Anterior enterocoele for example, could develop from unresected excess anterior peritoneum at the time of hysterectomy, and posterior enterocoele might arise from surgical procedures which changed the normally horizontal vaginal axis to vertical. Obstetric trauma to the upper and lower vagina also was a significant contributing factor to vaginal inversion or eversion.

Problems in diagnosis of enterocoele have been noted since

earliest times and Thomas (1885) remarked that unquestionably the greatest danger to the patient lay in diagnostic error. His point of view had great meaning when one considered that methods of excisional management current in those days, could produce damage to important viscera, and he cited colon and omentum. Misdiagnosis also meant risk of spontaneous rupture in an untreated enterocoele and "recurrence" following reparative surgery. He offered the following physical signs: "The vaginal swelling is supple, soft and yielding, decreasing in size with pressure and giving a sense of gurgling to the finger. It increases in size with straining and is resonant to percussion, yet easily reducible in the knee/chest position." Bueermann (1932) noted peristaltic waves coursing over the surface of the swelling following physical irritation and re-emphasized the plight of the patient with an incorrect diagnosis. No matter what method was used for diagnosis, many were not found until the cul-de-sac was explored during surgery and Hill (1957) reported only two enterocoeles diagnosed preoperatively in 505 Manchester procedures, yet eight were detected at surgery. Kinzel (1960) also emphasized the point that differentiation between enterocoele and rectocoele was sometimes difficult, and no matter what method was used in diagnosis, many would not be found until surgery was performed. The sac should always be opened during vaginal repair surgery. The usual presenting symptom was a vaginal swelling often without any physiological upset, although some complained of fullness in the rectum with unsatisfied defaecation and fewer of bladder symptoms. Usually symptoms had been present only for a short time, with a variable time before recurrence after previous surgery.

Sir Astley Cooper's description of a case was graphic. "A young woman aged twenty years, who had never had children, presented with a tumour projecting into the vagina. Placing herself in a recumbent posture, with the shoulders elevated, vaginal examination indicated a swelling a little above the external os, the size of which was that of a small billiard ball. It was situated at the posterior part of the vagina on the left, and not painful to the touch. When I compressed it, it readily passed away with upon directing her to cough it was reproduced. When I ordered her to place herself on her knees the swelling became very tense and much larger than before, when she coughed it dilated as any other hernia, but more forcibly. Having placed her again in the recumbent posture, I pressed the swelling entirely away by keeping the fingers about half a minute on the posterior part of the vagina then carrying the fingers high up in the vagina above the seat of the tumour near to the os uteri, having pushed the vagina toward the rectum, I directed her to cough and the tumour was not reproduced. Still pressing at the same part, I desired her to rise and so long as the pressure was sustained the hernia did not return, but almost immediately the fingers were removed the hernia became as large as before."

References to prophylaxis of enterocoele discuss what can be done during surgery to correct vaginal prolapse. Weed and Tyrone (1950) stated that posterior vaginal hernia subsequent to abdominal or vaginal hysterectomy could be prevented by proper inspection of the cul-de-sac, and its obliteration by approximation of the utero-sacrals. However, Campbell (1950) noted that some uterosacral ligaments were only thin folds of peritoneum and in an anatomical study, found the distal or sacral portion of the ligament was much weaker than the uterine. Pressure of difficult or repeated childbirth might injure this weak portion of the ligaments more, and hysterectomy removed the strong portion of the uterosacral ligaments, so stretching the distal portions even more. The truth of these facts was ignored and gynaecologists continued to advocate uterosacral ligament closure.

Read (1952) stated that strict adherence to the principles of repair would eliminate the so-called post-operative recurrent entero-coele which was in fact not recurrence but neglect. Waters and Glasser (1955) also believed there was no excuse for recurrent vault prolapse, because the specific anatomic defect responsible for pro-lapse of the vaginal vault, namely damage to the lateral supports of the vaginal fornices and walls, often was present already in the patient with a prolapsed uterus. Accordingly, repair of defects in these structures was essential for proper correction and prophylaxis of vault prolapse, by any route. One should recognize that entero-coele complicated nearly every case of prolapse in some degree and an unrepaired problem could initiate prolapse post-operatively. They advocated excision of redundant peritoneum followed by standard enterocoele repair, which meant excision of the sac and its obliteration, followed by high approximation of the uterosacral liga-ments. Kinzel (1961) advised exploring the cul-de-sac visually and digitally, and weak as the uterosacral ligaments seemed, never-theless their approximation helped prevent future herniation of small bowel between them. Nicholls (1972) included weight reduction, elimination of smoking and chronic constipation as important to prophylaxis of this problem.

Literature on the management of enterocoele is extensive under three major headings of prophylaxis, conservative management and operative correction. Prophylaxis has been discussed already. Conservative management has been to do entirely with a wide range of pessaries, and finally, proposed methods of operative correction have been legion, tackling the problem either by the vaginal route alone, by the abdominal route alone, or in combination. Surgical repair has been determined by many criteria including the need for future intercourse, the wish to have more children, whether or not a uterus is present, whether the surgeon prefers an abdominal or vaginal approach, and finally the presence of associated medical or surgical conditions. The principles of repair enunciated by Nicholls (1972) are the principles for repair of hernia anywhere in the body. The entity must be recognized as a hernia and the entire sac should be exposed, cleared from surrounding tissues, opened (herniotomy), obliterated by occluding the neck and then excised. Accessory repair should follow — herniorrhaphy or hernioplasty. The important feature to be achieved in any reconstruction is for the normal upper vaginal axis, previously the site of herniation, to now lie over a horizontal levator plate.

Anatomy of the Genital Tract Supports

There has been wide controversy, ranging over many aspects of the supporting anatomy of the genital tract, and although presently it is common belief that both the levator ani complex and pelvic cellular tissues have important complementary roles to play, nevertheless in the past there has been great argument as to which was the more important, and in particular how each exerted its effect on genital tract stability. These problems will be considered in terms of evolutionary anatomy, human anatomy, comparative anatomy, and functional anatomy.

Pelvic floor muscles which functioned as tail-movers in four footed mammals, became pelvic floor supporters in man with change to the erect attitude. Pubococcygeus dropped some of its coccygeal attachments in man to join its fellow from the opposite side in a median raphe, and this tendinous insertion between the tip of the coccyx and anus was a fibrous extension of the abbreviated caudal appendage. Studies in comparative anatomy make it seem certain that muscles which formed the pelvic diaphragm had undergone an evolutionary process for support as the upright position was assumed, and the caudal extremity abbreviated. Hernia through the vaginal outlet was minimised by this strong posterior segment, with a superimposed more mobile anterior segment and the vaginal slit running obliquely, so that force from above pressed the anterior segment against the posterior.

Evolutionary Anatomy

Elftman (1932) in a study on evolution of the pelvic floor in primates, commented upon necessary changes needed to adopt an upright posture. There were very fundamental differences between

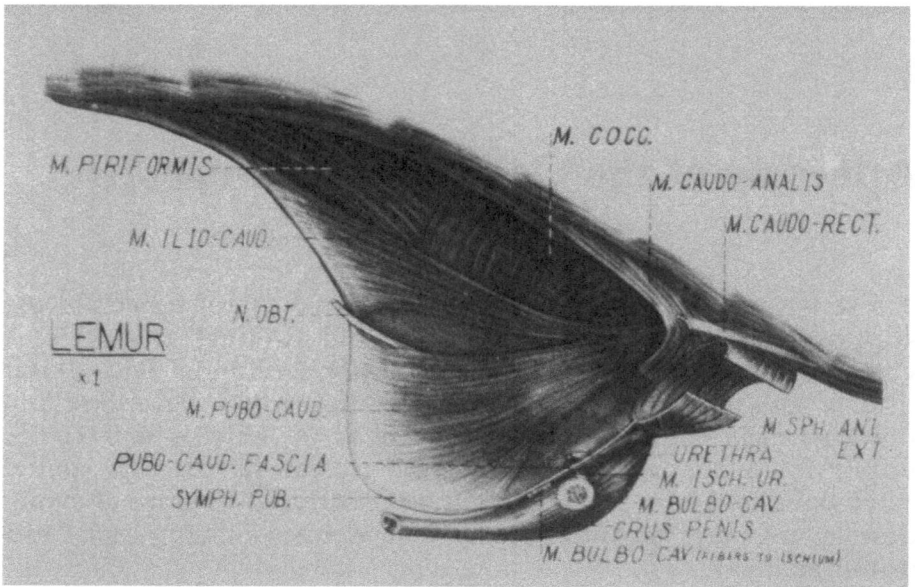

Figure 1. Sagittal section taken through the pelvis of the lemur in the sitting position. (From Elftman)

the pelvic floor of apes and man, and finding such differences had a direct bearing upon an understanding of man's evolution. The sitting position of the lemur could be compared roughly with that of a cat, in that visceral weight was supported, to a large extent by the abdominal wall and pelvic outlet, the latter frequently strengthened by the root of the tail (Fig. 1). The greatest strain on the outlet came when the lemur was climbing.

The only ape that could fairly be said to walk in an upright position in nature was the gibbon. Both chimpanzee and gorilla when on the ground, supported themselves on all fours, so the back of the animal was not horizontal, but sloped gently posteriorly, and only occasionally would the animal stand on its hind legs, and then its knees were bent. The upright position of man differed from that of any other primate in several crucial respects. He was the only primate doing the major portion of his work in an erect position, and as he walked, each jar was transmitted, although with diminished severity to the abdominal viscera, jouncing them toward the pelvic floor. The most obvious structure contributing to visceral support was the pelvic bone itself, the internal face of the ilium looked upward when the body was erect, so supported a good portion of the weight of the internal organs.

The chief muscles which aided in strengthening the pelvic floor could be considered in three groups, the first including levator ani with pyriformis, which closed the sacro-iliac foramen and reinforced coccygeus. The second group were the sphincter-cloacae muscles and the third, smooth muscle. Comparison of the bony pelvis in primates showed fundamental differences between ape and man. In the human a plane through the acetabuli and the centre of the sacro-iliac joints was almost perpendicular to the sacrum, but inclined slightly posteroventrally. A consequence of this arrangement could be seen in the pelvic outlet, the sacrum projecting caudally beyond the level of the ischial spine, and the coccyx curved so as to close the pelvic outlet more effectively (Fig. 2). In the gibbon the sacrum terminated far above the ischial spine (Fig. 4), but in both chimpanzee and gorilla, the sacrum and coccyx provided greater closure of the pelvic outlet than in the gibbon; yet in all these primates, the disposition of the sacrum and coccyx was such as to leave a weak area between the sacrum and anus (Fig. 5, 3). Also, the human sacrum was much wider.

In apes with the trunk erect, the symphysis pubis was almost vertical, whereas in man it inclined about 45° to the vertical, so enabling adjoining portions of the pubis and ischium to serve as partial visceral support. Again in man, the lumbar curve overhung the pelvis, forming a projection vertically above the pelvic outlet, and this bony arch seemed to locate the viscera more over the symphysis than over the pelvic outlet. Only after the bones and abdominal muscles had absorbed their share of the normal gravitational stresses, did the remaining burden fall on the outlet. The stresses here were not due mainly to viscera; but also to pressure created as mobile viscera jounced up and down. The abdominal muscles therefore had a great deal to do with equalization of intra-abdominal pressure.

Variability is one of the prime characteristics of pelvic musculature in man, and due to this factor, confusion has been rife, and argument waxed hot over descriptions of the human pelvic floor. However, there was an essential unanimity regarding the broad features of pelvic soft tissue structures. The pubococcygeus muscle in man, although varying considerably with respect to layers and other details, nevertheless constantly was regarded as one of the chief

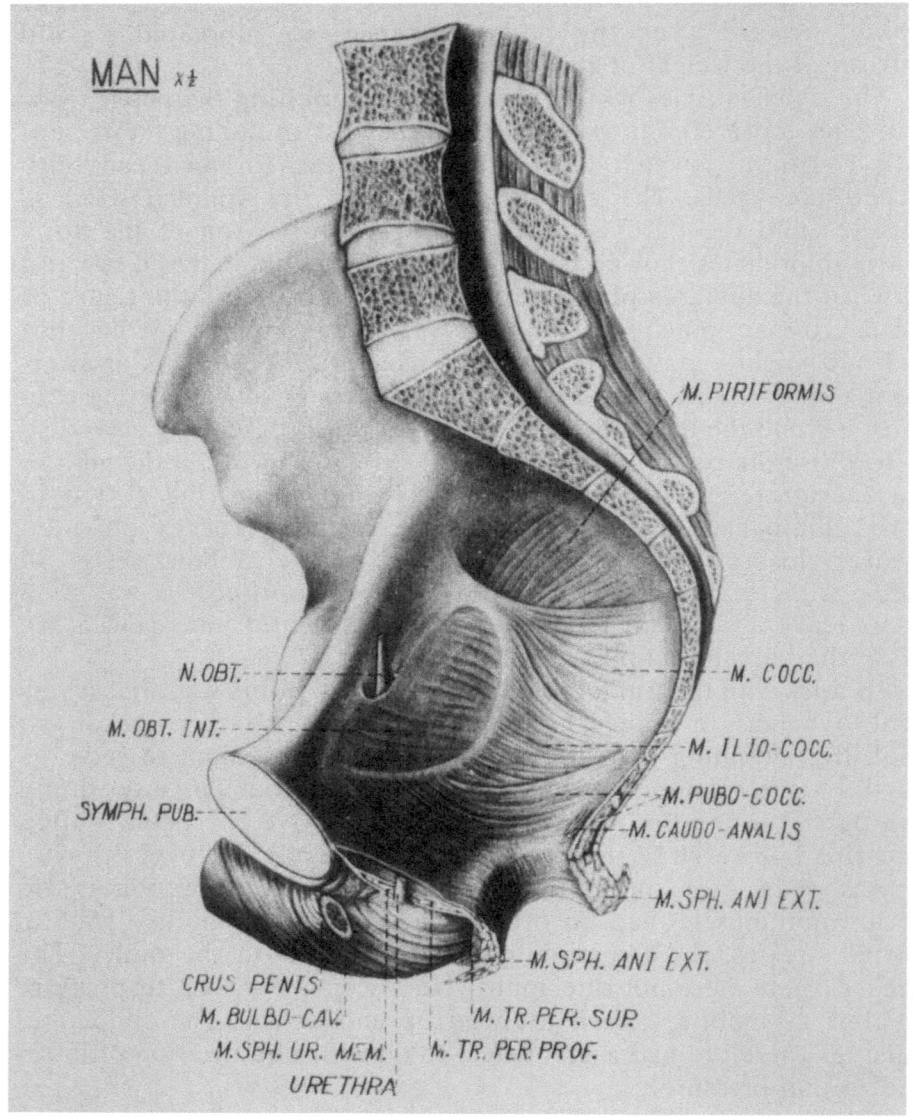

Figure 2. Midline sagittal section through a male human pelvis emphasizing the diminished pelvic outlet in comparison with the gibbon, chimpanzee and gorilla. (From Elftman)

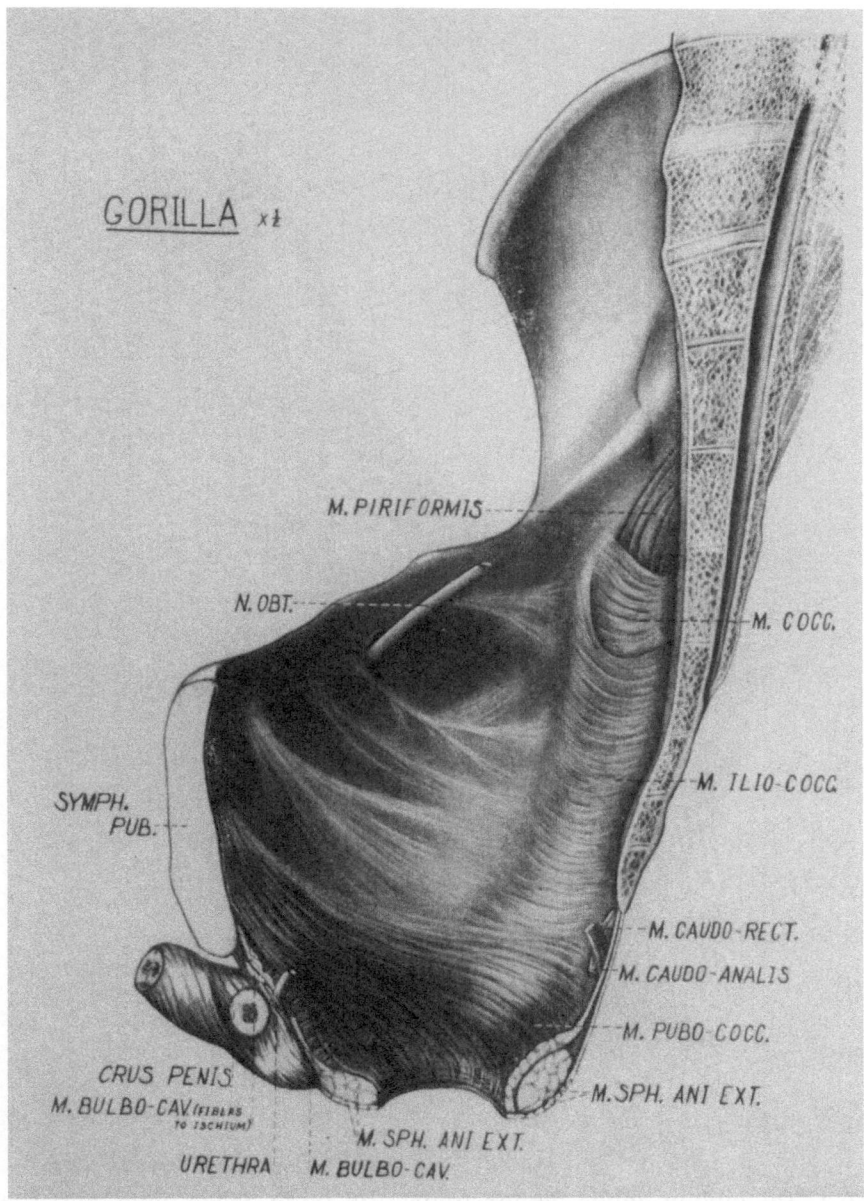

Figure 3. The gorilla pelvis showing a shorter pubic symphysis than in the chimpanzee and a narrower pelvic outlet. (From Elftman)

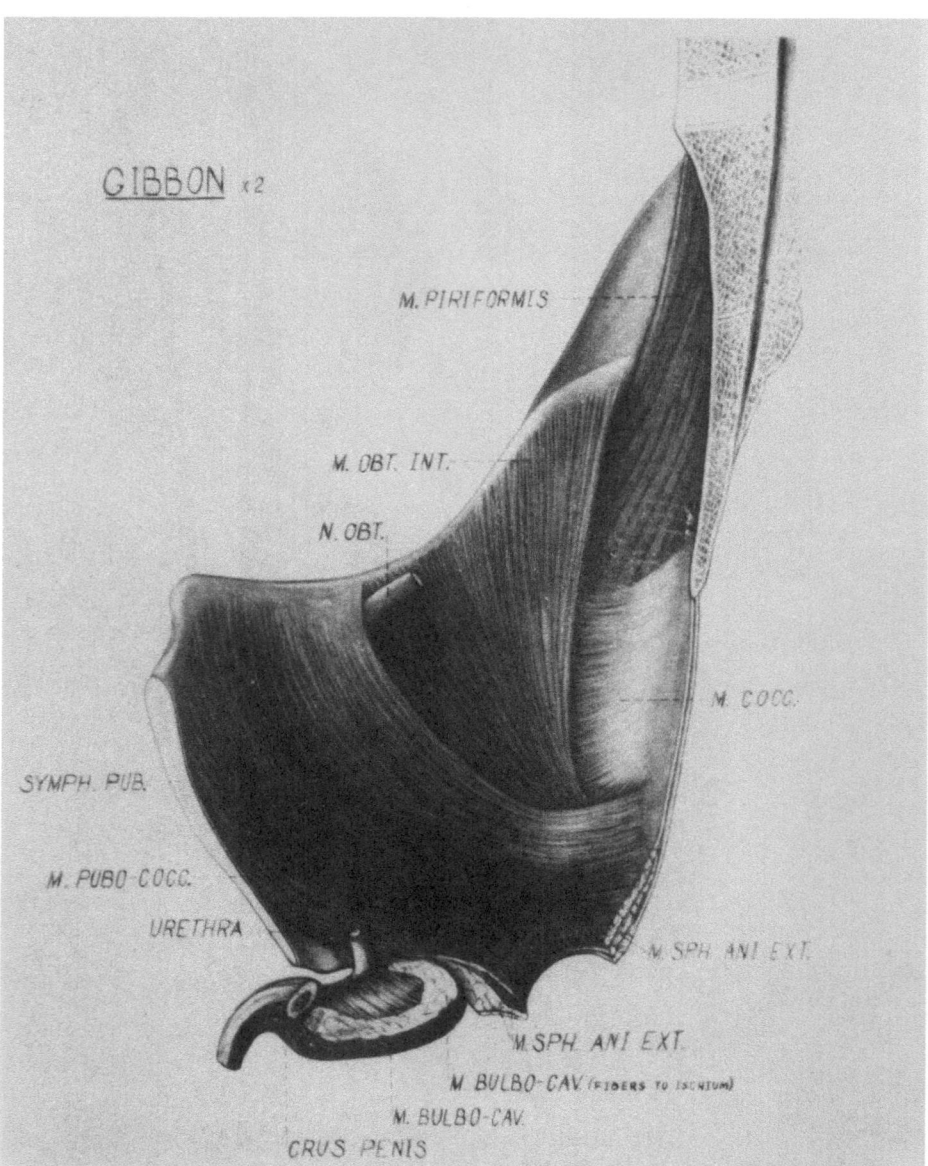

Figure 4. The gibbon pelvis demonstrating the wide pelvic outlet and the long symphysis pubis. (From Elftman)

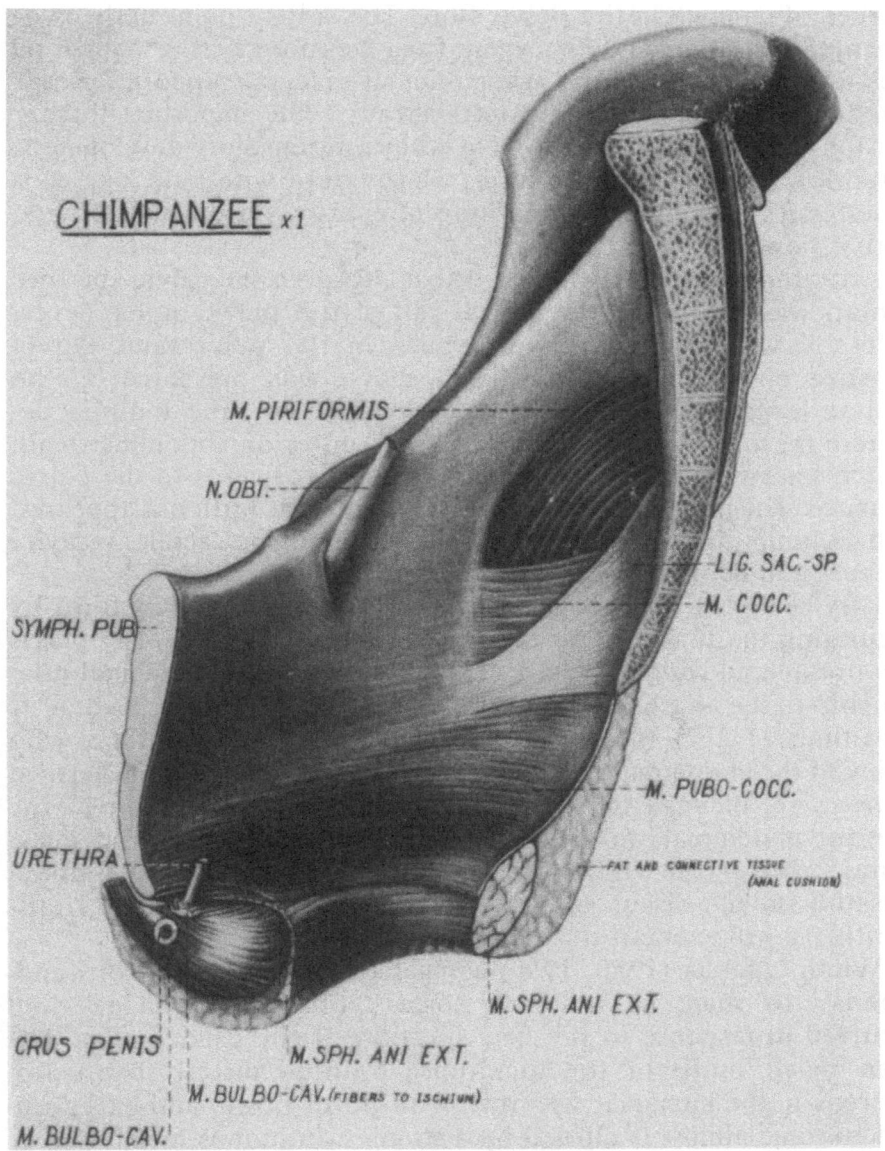

Figure 5. Sagittal section through the chimpanzee pelvis showing a pelvic outlet and symphysis pubis roughly midway between those of the gibbon and gorilla. (From Elftman)

sources of strength in the pelvic floor. The salient point in the evolution of levator ani and coccygeus from the monkey stage to that of
apes and man, was not the assumption of visceral support, for that
function these muscles performed already. The important feature
was loss of muscular development with compensatory development
of tendon and fascia — structures which could withstand long continued stresses without expenditure of energy yet did not provide
motive power.

Naunton Morgan (1948) noted that although the pelvic aperture
in man was situated at the lowest part of the pelvic outlet, nevertheless it was crowded forwards between the pubic rami. Direct
pressure on the pelvic floor from above was prevented by the
lumbar lordosis and the large sacral concavity. The lordosis de-
flected the initial thrust onto the lower anterior abdominal wall,
thence backward to the sacrum and finally forwards to the pelvic
aperture. The lumbar lordosis was not present at birth but appeared
with assumption of the erect posture and also the sacral concavity
increased in depth (see frontispiece).

Davies (1955) commented that man assumed the erect form by
angulating the lumbosacral area at the sacrum (Fig. 6). The pelvis
was not altered with this change, and bore the same horizontal relationship to the attached limbs as did the pelvis of a quadruped to its
hind limbs (Fig. 7). In a surgical aside, he remarked that those who
believed the abdominal and pelvic cavities were in the same vertical
plane, were inclined to suspend a prolapsed vaginal vault to the
anterior abdominal wall, although repeated failures and an occa-
sional enterocoele thereafter suggested that intra-abdominal
pressure on the viscus and its supports was increased by trans-
planting a pelvic organ into the abdominal cavity.

When Ulfelder (1956, 1960) compared pelvic anatomy of quadrupeds and man, he assumed some evolutionary changes had
occurred in response to the new situation of the pelvic outlet. The
open pelvic outlet of the quadruped pointed directly backward,
whereas in the human it was rotated to point down, and back, and
had become almost occluded by a strong continuous membrane of
muscle, tendon and bone. The pelvic diaphragm could be seen as a
tail, shortened and curved, then pulled across the outlet by muscles
which had become short, broad and attached to each other as well
as to the coccyx. The weak point of the outlet was reinforced by the
urogenital diaphragm, a structure seen only in man.

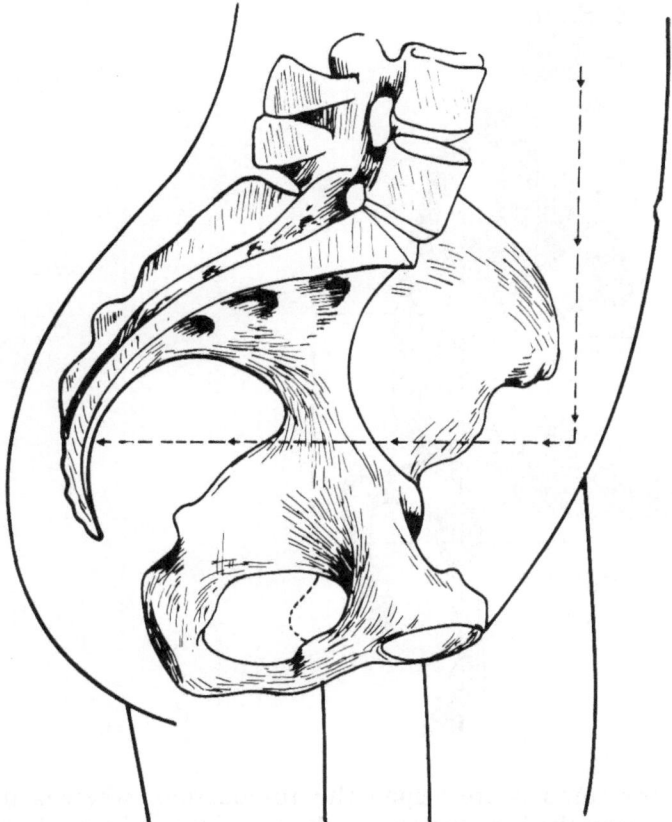

Figure 6. Pelvis of man with a vertical pelvic inlet and the bodies of S1 and S2 and the pubes are horizontal. The pelvic cavity is at right angles to the abdominal cavity due to the lumbosacral angulation. (From Davies)

In lower mammals, the symphysis is ischiopubic but with assumption of the erect attitude, the symphysis becomes pubic, and in birds, there is no direct bony apposition at all, the pubic bones being apart at the symphysis. With separation of the ischiopubic rami in man, the urogenital diaphragm has developed to support midline genital structures in the male — the bulb of the penis — so the membrane is developed less well in the female and also the vagina exits through it, so the vaginal outlet is a potential point of weakness in the supporting mechanism.

Assuming the erect posture has meant displacement of all the

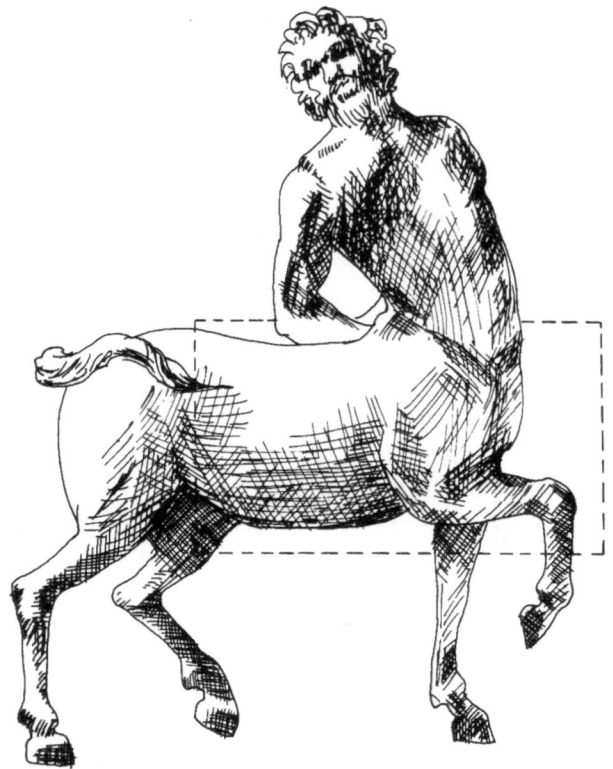

Figure 7. The Centaur's torso is erect upon the forequarters, whereas in man the torso is erect upon the hindquarters — the pelvis has the same horizontal relationship to the attached limbs. (From Davies)

iliac vasculature toward the sacrum, so the cardinal ligaments with the uterosacrals, extended from the cervix and upper vagina in a plane running posterolaterally and upward. The ligaments elevated the cervix as Mengert demonstrated, also they held it back in the concavity of the pelvis, so under normal circumstances the extent of forward and downward mobility of the cervix and vaginal apex was limited sharply. The sum of these effects was illustrated by the course of the birth canal, which began in the central axis as it did in the quadruped, but then pursued a gradual curve backward into the sacral cavity exactly as the lumbar curve of the vertebral column would dictate. At the level of the upper vagina the curve reversed itself and the canal thenceforth ran almost directly away from the sacrum, emerging at the forward margin of the pelvic outlet beneath the pubic arch. The combined effect of the ligaments holding the cervix back and the levator diaphragm displacing the vaginal orifice forward, was to impose a second curve on the human birth passage not seen in quadrupeds, and not directly the result of change from plantigrade to erect posture. This arrangement ensured that stresses from the abdominal cavity above, would be directed against structures strong enough to withstand them. Ulfelder agreeing with Elftman, considered that the marked forward curve of the lumbar spine, unique to man, placed a firm shelf beneath the abdominal viscera deflecting their weight against the strong muscles of the anterior abdominal wall. This curvature resulted in a junction of the pelvic ring with the vertical axis of the spine, at an angle far wider than 90°, an arrangement permitting the pubic arches and rectus abdominis muscles to continue support for the more anterior pelvic viscera.

The magnitude and frequency of pressure changes occurring within body cavities, meant that weakness in the surrounding bone or muscular shell would be exploited eventually, with protrusion of a sac. Potential weaknesses were at the point of exit of bowel, vagina and urethra through the pelvic floor, and the function of the urogenital diaphragm and sphincter ani muscles, was to buttress this area. Man's skeleton contributed to pelvic support chiefly by keeping as much bone as possible beneath the contents, so diverting much of the visceral burden off the pelvic floor, and at once the role of the levators became apparent. The supporting ligaments of the uterus acted as stays, concerned with preventing or minimising dislocation of the cervix from its normal position, so with the mechanism intact, the cervix would be found relatively immobile, well back in the pelvic basin, behind the anus, resting on the coccyx and the muscles and tendons which inserted into the sacrum and coccyx.

Human Anatomy

i) Pelvic Cellular Tissues

Much has been written about tissues which might contribute to genital tract support, with wide differences of opinion about the relative importance of pelvic connective tissues and levator ani, concerning their biological significance, physiological capacity and anatomical characteristics.

The condensations in the base of the broad ligaments were referred to first by Savage (1870), later described by Kocks (1880) as ligamenta cardinalia, and Mackenrodt (1895) termed them ligamentum transversum colli. Mackenrodt reported results from anatomical examinations made in the newborn, wherein he noted thick bandlike structures containing muscular elements which ran directly from the pelvic fascia to the vagina, rectum and bladder. Dorsally, he noted a mass of these fibres arranged like a band in the floor of the broad ligament yet distinctly separate from it, running into the cervix, — the ligamentum transversum colli — which began near the last lumbar vertebra, and extended to the side of the cervix where it attached. As the ilia developed, the ligament moved further laterally from the vertebral column, and finally lay in the transverse diameter with the uterine artery at its upper border. He described the utero-sacral ligaments, the pubovesicouterine ligaments and other bands which ran into the rectovaginal and vesicouterine septae, offering strong support to both rectum and bladder, whilst also serving to close the pelvic floor aperture. All bands were attached through the ligamentum transversum colli to the uterus which was the pivotal supporting structure, the bands supporting bladder and other pelvic organs also. These statements of Mackenrodt were accepted on face value without corroboration, and their adoption resulted not only in the development of a nomenclature, but also hypotheses to explain the mechanism of prolapse. Finally, operations were developed to cure the condition, accepting as fundamental the existence of the ligaments and fascia, as Mackenrodt had described them.

Even at that time some held different beliefs. Winter (1896) stated, "The uterus can be drawn against the symphysis, pushed into the hollow of the sacrum, shoved against the side wall of the pelvis, the fundus may be raised almost to the navel and the cervix can be pulled down to the vaginal orifice without causing pain. It is obvious therefore that peritoneum and so-called ligaments cannot have any real influence on the fastening of the uterus." Waldeyer (1899) remarked, "It is clear that all those structures which are related to the uterus help to hold it in place. Prime importance is given now to one and later to another. In my opinion it is the vagina and perineum, and next the blood vessels with their firm connective tissue sheaths which should be named as of first importance."

Anatomical opinion to this time had been largely European and widely accepted, particularly the work of Mackenrodt; but in 1902, Keith changed the whole picture around, and began a controversy which has persisted to this day, when he made the following statement, "It has been customary to regard fasciae as separate structures forming distinct sheets with devious and complex courses. It is possible by dissection, to prepare and display them according to accepted descriptions; but the structures so displayed are artificial and not the true structures with which the surgeon or physician has to deal." Derry (1907) commented that "the viscera therefore were simply invested by remains of the tissue in which they were originally developed, and the same applied to vessels which supplied them. The tissue was condensed in places to form definite ensheathing layers, particularly in the neighborhood of the vagina and lower part of the uterus. Any attempt to make such layers definitive was not only artificial; but made the description unnecessarily complex and confusing, for the simple reason that those layers although well marked in the regions named, and also around the rectum, passed gradually into the general mass of subperitoneal tissue which filled the whole pelvic cavity and then were traceable no longer."

The continuation of the ligamentum transversum colli from the pelvic fascia into the vagina was termed "paracolpos" by Fothergill (1907) and it was his view that the uterus, vagina and bladder were kept in place mainly by the lateral combination of unstriated muscle and connective tissue derived from pelvic fascia. So the pelvic organs were propped up partly from below, and partly suspended, but also he realised that extended experience in gynaecological surgery showed this accepted teaching was unsatisfactory. Extreme laxity of the perineal muscles could exist without genital tract descent, and in parous women often it was difficult or impossible to recognize the margin of the levator ani muscle. Often the vagina itself descended without seriously affecting the position of the other pelvic viscera, for cystocoele alone, rectocoele alone or the two combined, could be observed with a normally situated uterus. Therefore, genital tract support from below was irrelevant and similar observations pointed to the conclusion that suspension by uterine ligaments was even less important. He concluded that "the surgeon who looks at and handles so-called uterine ligaments day after day, with an ever waning sense of their mechanical importance, becomes convinced that structures credited with pelvic organ support do not perform those functions ascribed to them, except in a very minor degree." During vaginal hysterectomy, the uterus remained fixed solely by tissues known as parametrium and until this was divided on either side, the organ remained supported as completely as before. He concluded "that vessels and other structures with sheaths or fascial coverings lying to either side of the uterus below the broad ligament and above the fornices, were the structures supporting the uterus." Perivascular sheaths attached the pelvic organs to the sides of the funnel-shaped diaphragm, and without this firm attachment the pelvic viscera would "slip through its lower opening like sand through an hour-glass." Loosening this attachment must be regarded as the constant and essential factor in the cause of genital prolapse. Providing organs remained firmly attached above, enlargement of the outlet would not make them descend, and as further clinical evidence favouring this view, he cited patients in whom a well-developed prolapse had been cured by the onset of pelvic cellulitis. Successful vaginal hysterectomy performed for prolapse, depended upon effective measures to secure good union between right and left parametrial tissues. Fothergill stated categorically that the pelvic diaphragm did not support pelvic organs by its muscular action or by virtue of its shape, unless they were firmly attached to its sloping lateral walls, the attachment being accomplished by the fibrous sheaths of bloodvessels and accompanying structures which supplied the pelvic viscera. Classic descriptions of pelvic fascia should be discarded he advised, and fascia regarded as sheaths of muscles, vessels and viscera. The one constant cause of prolapse was relaxation of the perivascular sheaths!! And so the case for pre-eminence of pelvic cellular tissues as upper genital tract supports was advanced. Fothergill was unimpressed with the levator ani complex, believing its sole importance lay in a support role because of genital tract attachment to it, by paracolpos and parametrium. Naturally he put the view that attention to these tissues was the key to corrective surgery for prolapse.

Halban and Tandler (1907) held opposite opinions to Fothergill, contending that pelvic floor muscles were the main support for the pelvic viscera. An important but subsidiary role was attributed to the "fascia endopelvina", a fascial sheath which surrounded the uterus, bladder and rectum, fixing them in their normal position, whilst permitting free mobility.

It was Thelander's view (1922) that providing the vagina stayed in its normal position, intra-abdominal pressure closed it by pressing the anterior and posterior walls together, so uterine prolapse would be infrequent. The determining factor in the production of prolapse was the integrity of structures supporting the vaginal vault, and of these he regarded the uterosacral ligaments as most important. Like Mackenrodt, he considered the round ligaments contributed nothing, for their lack of tension always was notable, and even if they could contract, the only effect would be to increase anteversion of the uterine fundus. He believed the main function of the round ligaments, judging from the multiplicity of surgical procedures in which they were involved, was "to offer a fairly safe reason for the exercise of surgical ingenuity and enterprise." At laparotomy he resected a portion of both round ligaments near their uterine ends, brought the uterus into retroversion and filled the vesicouterine space with intestine; but upon discharge from hospital the uterus was found in its original position of anteversion. Despite evidence such as this, which indicated clearly that the round ligaments played no effective role in uterine support, nevertheless they continued to figure prominently in many operative procedures designed to cure or ameliorate prolapse. Even at present, some of this thinking still is put forward and acted upon. Despite the great authority of Mackenrodt and Fothergill and their pronouncements upon the importance of the pelvic cellular tissues, during the nineteen thirties many careful investigations of these tissues were reported which refuted these widely held opinions. Hand in hand with these reports other anatomical factors were suggested as important to genital tract support.

Goff (1931) in a careful histological scrutiny of a normal nulliparous pelvis, could not find any tissue in the walls of the vagina, urethra, bladder or rectum which logically could be called fascia.

There was no fascia between the anterior vaginal wall and urethra, although a thin layer of areolar tissue was present between the anterior vaginal wall and bladder. A similar layer of areolar tissue occurred between the posterior vaginal wall and rectum. The areolar character of this tissue made it impossible to dissect as an individual layer, so clearly it could not be utilised in vaginal plastic procedures. If used at all in surgery, it would be in conjunction with the overlying vaginal wall, and apparently many gynaecologists had applied the term "fascia" to the muscular coat of the vaginal wall situated just below the mucosa, since it resembled a layer of dense fascia in its gross appearance.

Koster (1933) critically reviewed the value of "ligaments" as uterine supports, concluding that they could not be very effectual. From autopsy material in multiparous females, he examined the structure of the vesicovaginal and rectovaginal septae microscopically, but found no evidence of a fascial structure comparable to that described by Mackenrodt. Similarly in operative material, he could not find fascia in either septum but only loose areolar tissue without supportive or restraining value. In further autopsy studies, tissues related to the uterine arteries in their course from the internal iliac artery to the uterus were investigated, looking for the ligaments of Mackenrodt, and here again the result was negative. Sections from the rectovaginal septum beginning above and running down to the perineum, showed the vaginal wall separated from the rectum only by loose areolar connective tissue, and nowhere was fascial tissue detected. His findings confirmed Goff's work and he concluded that there was no well-formed, dense fascial tissue in either the rectovaginal or vesicovaginal septum. In the adult, tissue related to the uterine artery between the internal iliac artery and the junction of the cervix and body of the uterus, was not comparable to the ligamentous structure known as the "cardinal ligament". Microscopically no such tissue was demonstrable, suggesting that the prominence given to Mackenrodt's ligament as a uterine support was unwarranted, and operations to cure prolapse by shortening or plicating these ligaments, advocated by Nyulasy (1921), could have no rational basis. Accordingly, Koster proposed that in seeking explanations for the development of prolapse and its cure, the so-called ligaments should be excluded from consideration.

Sears (1935) removed tissue from the anterior and posterior fascial planes of the vagina at operation. The anterior wall specimens showed many bands of muscle, bloodvessels of varying size, areolar tissue and fibro-elastic connective tissue. Similarly, specimens from the posterior wall, although containing some muscle fibres, were composed principally of rather compact connective tissue with strands of interspersed fibro-elastic tissue. Over the rectal aspect of the posterior wall, the density of connective tissue in the specimen was increased. Although definite, the broad firm sheets of tissue which could be dissected from the vaginal walls were not composed of fascia alone but of muscle, connective tissue and compact strands of fibro-elastic tissue, the latter intermingling with muscle fibres and appearing as definite broad strands along the surface of the vaginal musculature. The muscle was more in evidence in sections from the anterior wall. These contributions showed clearly the poor quality of so-called pelvic ligaments and pointed to the futility of employing them in proposed surgical repair of genital prolapse.

No doubt the primacy of pelvic cellular tissue in arguments about genital tract support would have faded gradually had it not been for the work of Mengert (1936) who made a classic contribution to pelvic floor anatomy by quantitative evaluation of the relative importance of each means by which the uterus could be retained in the pelvis. Legendre and Bastien (1858) first had reported information gained by traction on the uterus of a cadaver, and Mengert repeated their work. He used 8 cadavers all in a state of normal nutrition at death, with apparently normal pelvic organs and most importantly, no evidence of genital prolapse. Each cadaver lay supine with a tenaculum on each lip of the cervix, attached to a string with a 1 Kgm weight passing over a pulley at the foot of the table. A metre bar on the table parallel to the string between the legs of the cadaver measured the descent of the uterus accurately as successive structures were severed, and paired structures attached to the uterus were cut in varying sequences, eight pairs of structures being recognized.

1) Round ligaments.
2) Ovarian and infundibulopelvic ligaments.
3) Upper third of broad ligaments.
4) Lower two-thirds of broad ligaments.
5) Upper third of paravaginal tissues.
6) Middle third of paravaginal tissues.
7) Uterosacral ligaments.
8) Pubocervical ligaments.

In addition, pelvic floor musculature was considered as a possible uterine support, and in 2 subjects the vagina was detached from the cervix by circumcision early in the experiment. Obviously this procedure eliminated the paravaginal tissues from consideration in those 2 subjects. The results were most interesting. Division of the round, ovarian, infundibulopelvic, and upper portion of the broad ligament did not affect uterine position. In 3 cadavers, when all parametrial and paravaginal tissues were severed and the round ligaments left intact, the cervix prolapsed through the introitus without even tensing them. The uterosacral ligaments furnished a small amount of support, explainable by their close anatomical connection to parametrial tissues. The pubocervical ligaments played a negligible role. The pelvic diaphragm and pelvic floor remained intact in all 8 cadavers and in no instance interfered with uterine descent, so Mengert doubted whether the pelvic floor afforded any uterine support. Division of parametrial and paravaginal tissues comprising the lower two-thirds of paravaginal structures, allowed an average uterine descent of 10.5 cms. Marked descent of the uterus amounting to actual prolapse never occurred so long as any part of the upper two-thirds of the paravaginal and/or lower two-thirds of the parametrial tissues was intact. In three instances in which all uterine connective tissues above the vagina were severed, notable descent did not occur, indicating that the vagina not only had its own support but could maintain the uterus as well. Parametrial and paravaginal tissues were identical anatomical structures, the latter being merely continuations of the former and separate terms were used just for greater exactness in localization.

As indicated, the work of Mengert re-established the important supportive role of the parametrial tissues and denigrated the role of the levator complex. It was of course fashionable at that time — and indeed still is in some present texts — to depict the genital tract poised over the levator hiatus and about to slip through this obvious defect, prevented only by the parametrial tissues. Several more important papers at that time promoted the views of Mengert.

Power (1939) reviewed anatomical descriptions of uterine supporting tissues, and noted that Moritz (1913) had denied Mackenrodt's ligaments to be separate structures, maintaining they were simple pelvic areolar tissue strengthened by perivascular sheaths. Power observed smooth muscle tissue lying between the pelvic peritoneum and the upper superior surface of levator ani arranged as a series of bundles radiating from the uterus at the level of the internal os. He divided them into three groups — anterior, lateral and posterior, and further subdivided each group into smaller subgroups of fibres. He believed this smooth or unstriated muscle was particularly important since it had the ability to maintain tension or tonus and withstand extension or stretching which could not be tolerated by mere fascia. Also, if its power of maintaining tonus had been lessened for nutritional or mechanical reasons, it would be a less efficient supporting structure than fascia. Finally he commented that smooth muscle had the property of maintaining the same tonic force within narrow limits irrespective of the degree of stretch to which it was subjected, until the limit of elasticity was reached, then it behaved as an inactive fascial tissue. He concluded that muscle tissue was found precisely in regions where one might expect to find it, and where it was necessary to permit considerable dilatation, contraction or movement of organs, all the while maintaining some degree of control of movement of these organs independently, and in relation to one another.

Curtis et al. (1940) describing the anatomy of the uterine vessels, commented that the walls of the vascular sheath with its contained vessels appeared as a considerable mass continuous with the subjacent heavy ligament, and it was customary to consider the whole assemblage as the cardinal or Mackenrodt ligament. From the top of the vascular compartment downward, the parametrium thickened and consisted of two definite layers, the posterior layer being continuous with the uterosacral ligament, blending in turn with the more dense portion of the cardinal ligament so an intimate connection was effected (Fig. 8). An explanation for valuable uterine support obtained by suturing the uterosacral ligaments together with silk now was apparent. The uterosacral formed the medial border of and integrated with the Mackenrodt ligament, so division of it and the adjacent parametrium released uterine fixation and support proportional to the extent to which the scissors cut laterally and transversely through those tissues. Removal of the uterosacral ligaments meant the heavier adjacent structure with which they were continuous, remained on each side and this was Mackenrodt tissue which included the definite fibrous sheath which covered the vessels. The vascular core contained uterine artery and veins placed essentially transversely in the broad ligament base and the entire mass constituting Mackenrodt tissue spread tentlike laterally toward

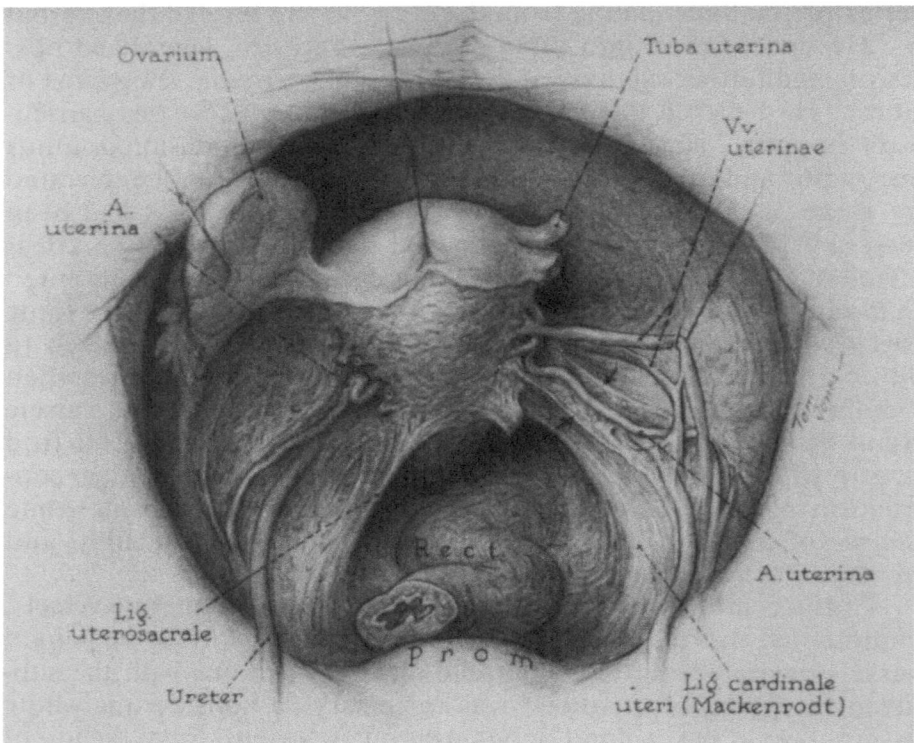

Figure 8. Diagram showing vascular and ligamentous structures which lie within the broad ligament. The arrows indicate the two layers of the broad ligament. (From Curtis et al.)

the pelvic wall, becoming attached to the fascia which overlay the obturator muscle and the superior fascia of the pelvic diaphragm. Also, it merged medially and inferiorly into the uterovaginal and vesical fascial envelopes, and integrated posteriorly with the uterosacral (Fig. 9). The authors agreed with Mengert whose experiments showed that the Mackenrodt ligaments with their perivaginal continuations were the chief uterine supports.

Having apparently solved the enigma of the Mackenrodt tissue and assigning to it, its proper supportive role, investigators now turned their attention to the rectovaginal septum and the pouch of Douglas, believing that defects in these anatomical structures might well play a role in the development of genital prolapse, particularly enterocoele. Tobin and Benjamin (1945) realised that opposing

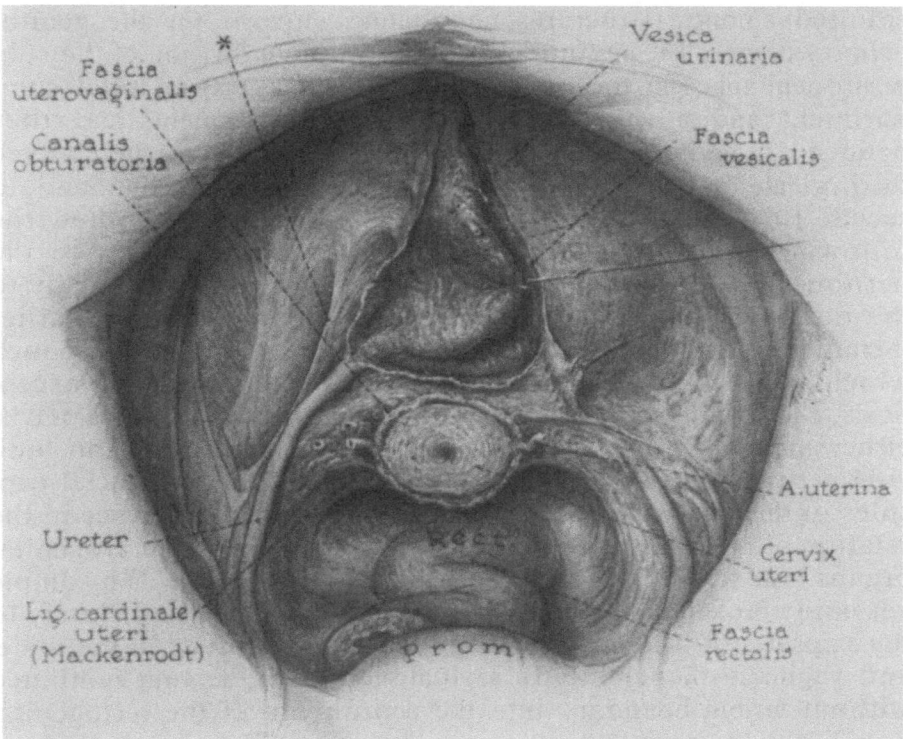

Figure 9. Diagram depicting basal structures in the broad ligament and the relation between Mackenrodt tissue and adjacent important structures. (From Curtis et al.)

views concerning the embryological origin of Denonvilliers fascia, from mesenchyme (Wesson, 1923) or peritoneum (Cuneo and Veau, 1899) appeared due to differences in concept of tissues which made up peritoneum. Their studies indicated that the only part of Denonvilliers fascia derived from peritoneum was the fibrous membrane remaining following obliteration of the cavity in the pelvic cul-de-sac, and contrary to Wesson's opinion, that peritoneum reverted to undifferentiated tissue in the embryo, they found the fibrous membrane derived from the peritoneum was present in all the adult specimens and its origin could be traced in the variously aged embryos and foetuses studied.

Uhlenhuth et al. (1948) regarded the rectovaginal septum as especially important, since it separated rectum from vagina and could be counted amongst structures constituting support for the genito-urinary organs. The septum effected a complete division of the sub-peritoneal space in the pelvic cavity, into a dorsal or rectal com-partment and a ventral or urogenital compartment, and they believed a peritoneal origin explained the anatomy best. Even during late intrauterine life, the urogenital pouch continued to recede from the rectogenital space and accordingly they drew the following conclusions: In the female it attached cranially to the peritoneum at the bottom of the pouch of Douglas and caudally to the dorsal surface of the vagina. It resulted from fusion in earlier intrauterine life between the front and back walls of the pouch which extended originally to the pelvic floor, and with few excep-tions, the septum could be demonstrated clearly in an adult pelvis, either male or female. In most instances the septum was an indi-vidual structure, additional to and independent of the fascial cap-sules of the adjacent viscera. There was a constant difference in the relation of the septum to the capsules of the rectum and urogenital organs. The septum was separated from the rectal capsule by ample yet easily broken down loose areolar tissue; but adhered closely to the capsules of bladder, seminal vesicles and prostate in the male, and vagina in the female. In sagittal section the septum continued without visible boundary into the peritoneum of the rectogenital pouch and its surface texture was entirely different from that of adjacent fascial membranes, being evenly membranous and glis-tening, sometimes showing a faintly greenish colour — the duck egg blue of the late Sir Charles Read. Nicholls and Milley (1970) noted the presence of a thin yet firm membrane which obstructed passage of the surgeon's finger at the vaginal apex, during dissection of the rectovaginal space. They repeated the work of Uhlenhuth et al and found the septum present in 34 of 36 female cadavers, with the same superior and inferior attachments (Fig. 10). The persistent attachment to the posterior vaginal wall helped explain the reluctance to accept this tissue as an entity. Approximating the cut edges of the septum during posterior colpoperineorrhaphy, directed the vagina toward the sacrum by increasing tension on the lateral septal attachments — this tended to replace the vagina in its correct position with a horizontal axis.

Anatomical reports returned at this time to the old riddle of the pelvic cellular tissues, with two important contributions. Campbell (1950) stated that by virtue of location, course, attachment, and

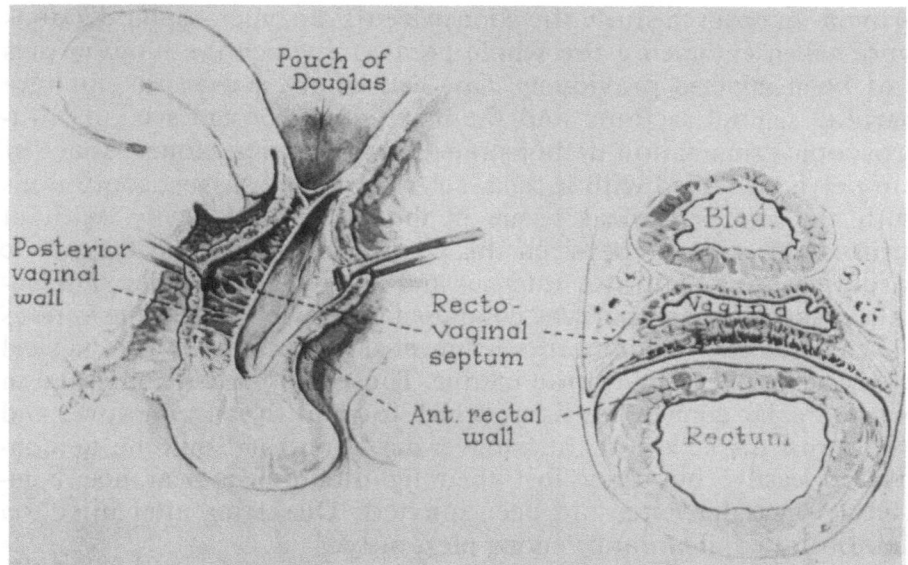

Figure 10. The rectovaginal septum seen extending between the floor of the pouch of Douglas and the perineal body. The septum has a posterolateral curve and adheres to the posterior vaginal wall rather than to the rectum. (From Nicholls and Milley)

fibromuscular components, the uterosacral ligaments should be regarded as important factors in holding the cervix upward and backward, yet he found that the matrix of the intermediate and posterior or sacral thirds of these ligaments was composed mainly of loose connective tissue, and concluded that they should not be credited with undue supportive value. The uterine end was quite often well developed; but the weak, insignificant development of the posterior aspect was noteworthy. He mentioned the old adage that a chain was no stronger than its weakest link, so the supportive action of the posterior third of the ligament was certainly questionable. Berglas and Rubin (1953) correlated much past information and reached certain conclusions. They conducted histologic studies of pelvic connective tissue and showed, like Koster, that there was no anatomical basis for assuming pelvic organs were supported by connective tissue structures. Ligamentous condensations as such did not exist, and the fixation of pelvic connective tissue to the pelvic walls put forward forcefully by Fothergill, could not be proven. In order to study the connective tissue, microscopic sections were taken embracing the whole pelvis, in which the bloodvessels had been injected previously. One half of the pelvis was cut into parallel sagittal sections and the other, into coronal sections. Microscopic examination demonstrated that the subperitoneal space of the pelvis was filled with loose areolar connective tissue, continuous with the retroperitoneal tissue of the abdominal cavity, without intimate attachment between this connective tissue and the pelvic fascia covering obturator internus and the levator muscles. The so-called cardinal ligament was composed chiefly of the uterine venous plexus, and the vesicouterine ligament corresponded to the vesical plexus as it merged with the uterine. These plexi were embedded in loose areolar connective tissue which formed their framework, and with gross dissection in the cadaver the ligaments could be demonstrated easily; but they lost their ligamentous appearance completely once the veins had been injected. Dissecting after injection demonstrated abundant venous plexi only.

Histologic sections showed the cardinal ligament did not exist, and instead, bloodvessels were found in loose areolar connective tissue. Dense fibrous tissue with fibres grouped into large bundles as one might expect in ligamentous structures could not be found anywhere in these areas. Traction on the so-called Mackenrodt tissue led to complete compression of the lumina of the venous plexi, their walls imparting the palpatory sensation of a band-like condensation — the so-called "chicken wire effect", but a ligament could not be palpated on the other side which was not under tension. Fixation of parametrium to the pelvic wall by a connective tissue attachment to pelvic fascia did not exist and the commonly assumed fixation could be explained by the fact that arteries and veins embedded in areolar connective tissue of the parametrium were continuous with the main venous and arterial channels situated on the lateral pelvic wall. The work of Mengert, and similar observations made during vaginal hysterectomy, indicated that during traction the bloodvessels and connective tissue prevented wide movements and downward displacement of the uterus and vagina; but this would not prove the effectiveness of those structures in maintaining normal uterine position in the living female under normal conditions. Parametrial reaction to the constant effect of intra-abdominal pressure was elongation and hypertrophy, and whilst parametrial and paravaginal tissues could resist traction exerted on the cervix during vaginal hysterectomy and in the cadaver experiments of Mengert, they would not withstand the prolonged action of intra-abdominal pressure, and elongated accordingly.

To suggest that relaxation and elongation of these connective tissues were aetiological factors in visceral displacement was to reverse the order of cause and effect. The names parametrial, para-vesical, vesicovaginal and rectovaginal should serve merely to designate topographic location and distribution of subperitoneal connective tissue, for the arrangement of pelvic connective tissue and texture was essentially the same in all those different areas. Ret-roperitoneal connective tissue is the same throughout the pelvis and does not deserve special designations in relation to the uterus. This most important paper placed pelvic cellular tissues into their proper perspective and laid the Mackenrodt myth. It simply restated the views of Derry (1907). It is now widely appreciated that the so-called ligaments are connective tissue condensations about the vas-cular pedicles travelling from the lateral pelvic wall to the uterus, cervix and vagina. Relaxation and elongation of these tissues, once believed to be the cause of genital prolapse, is now considered to be produced by the developing prolapse — which is a complete reversal of past thinking.

ii) Levator Ani

With adoption of the erect attitude by man, muscles used by four-footed animals to depress and move the tail laterally, changed their function to become supporters of the pelvic floor, and are grouped together by anatomists as the levator ani complex. There has been misunderstanding of the muscles of the pelvic floor, and in partic-ular confusion about nomenclature, since earliest descriptions. Orig-inally the levator muscle was described by Vesalius, and Holl (1897) temed the fibres which slung the lower rectum, the puborectalis. Thompson (1899) described the pelvic floor as a compact mass in which two distinct layers of muscles could be recognized, with arrangement and function in striking contrast. The upper layer formed a more or less complete pelvic diaphragm, whereas the lower, as if designed for purposes of control, formed sphincters for openings of canals which perforated the floor to reach the exterior. The two layers were different functionally and morphologically.

Muscles of the upper layer with their aponeuroses formed the pelvic diaphragm, a funnel-shaped sling which encircled the pelvic viscera, deep behind, shallow in front, widely open above and with a narrow outlet below.

Dickinson (1899) described the muscle as horse-shoe-shaped and its ends were attached behind the pubes, whilst the urethra, vagina and anal canal passed between its right and left sides.

The component parts of the muscle, pubococcygeus, iliococcygeus, ischiococcygeus, coccygeus and puborectalis have long been standard nomenclature, yet careful dissection of the muscle has indicated a more complex anatomy than this simple description. Gray's Anatomy described the muscle as broad and thin, attached to the inner surface of the lateral pelvic wall, and uniting with its fellow from the opposite side to form the greater part of the floor of the pelvic cavity. Anteriorly, it arose from the pelvic surface of the pubic body lateral to the symphysis, and posteriorly from the inner surface of the ischial spine. Between these two points it took origin by the so-called "white line". from the obturator fascia. From these origins the fibres passed medially with varying degrees of obliquity, the most anterior fibres sweeping backward and down across the side of the prostate in the male to insert into the perineal body, and in the female they crossed the side of the vagina to insert into the side of that structure. Succeeding fibres passed back and down across the side of the prostate and upper anal canal to turn medially at the anorectal flexure, becoming continuous with corresponding fibres from the opposite side, a number being lost in the wall of the anal canal — the puborectalis. Remaining fibres inserted into the last two pieces of the coccyx, and a median fibrous raphe stretching between the coccyx and the anorectal flexure. Nerve supply was from the 4th sacral nerve, and a branch which arose from either the perineal or inferior haemorrhoidal division of the pudendal nerve. The muscle constricted the lower end of the rectum and vagina, steadied the perineal body and formed a diaphragm supporting pelvic viscera — the pelvic diaphragm — which opposed the downward thrust of intra-abdominal pressure.

Goff (1928) considered the muscle composed of three separate flat segments, a dividing line across the muscle on a level with the junction of the superior pubic ramus and ilium separating those fibres which inserted into the coccyx and posterior portion of the fibrous raphe, from those passing to the anterior part of the raphe and rectum. Each part was supplied by a separate nerve, and comparative anatomical studies indicated that the posterior levator — the iliococcygeus — was quite distinct from the anterior. Probably the anterior levator consisted of two morphologically separate muscles, the first, pubococcygeus which arose from the pubis and anterior part of the "white line" to insert into the median raphe, and the second, puborectalis, situated beneath it consisting of fibres arising from the pubis which inserted mainly into the rectum; but others passed between the rectum and vagina to insert into the perineal body (Fibres of Luschka).

According to Sturmdorf (1919), "pubococcygeus and puborectalis had a line of origin extending 1½ inches on either side of the posterior surface of the pubic symphysis, equalling in width the average sternomastoid muscle, being twice as thick as the diaphragm and weighing one quarter as much as the external oblique, and altogether presented a muscular support exceeding that which guards the inguinal ring. The median borders of this muscle were palpable plainly through the lateral vaginal wall, ½" or less behind the plane of the hymen, to form a V-shaped interspace embracing the introitus under the pubic arch — "the hiatus genitalis".

Lawson (1974) made a detailed study of pelvic floor muscles in neonatal and infant pelves which indicated a subdivision into two groups, with a functional application. Since the accounts of Holl (1897) and Thompson (1899) the muscles had been divided on comparative anatomical grounds. Pubococcygeus included muscle arising from the pubis, either directly from the body or indirectly from the superior ramus via the white line. Iliococcygeus included fibres from the remainder of the white line, and thus indirectly via the attachment of the obturator fascia to the superior ramus of the ilium and from the medial aspect of the ischium. Ischiococcygeus or coccygeus derived from the tip and posterior border of the ischial spine. Though the plane between iliococcygeus and coccygeus was clear, the separation of pubococcygeus from iliococcygeus was based on an imaginary line running from the anterior edge of the ischial tuberosity to the junction of the superior pubic ramus with that of the ilium. However, Lawson's dissection showed a clear plane of cleavage between muscles which arose from the body of the pubis, and those arising from the white line. Studying muscle insertion, he noted that muscles from the pubic body inserted either directly into or provided a sling for structures associated intimately with pelvic viscera — "the pubovisceral group". On the other hand, muscles from the white line formed a continuous sheet inserting predominantly into skeletal structures, namely the lower sacral and coccygeal vertebrae, and also coccygeus fanned to insert into the sacrum and coccyx lateral to the sacral foraminae. All these muscles were termed "the diaphragmatic group". The levator complex sloped medially, down and forward to form a gutter in which lay the rectum. Anteriorly the viscera passed through the space in front of this arch and behind the pubis, supported by pubovisceral muscles which extended from the pubis to individual viscera, filling the lateral spaces and performing a secondary diaphragmatic role. The pubovisceral group arose from a curved origin, convex upward from the back of the pubis, and at the origin, made up two well-defined layers, upper and lower; but with differing male and female viscera, constituent muscles and attachments varied. In the male, the upper layer constituted the major component, termed puboanalis. The more anterior fibres inserted into the circumference of the anal canal, whilst the more posterior spiralled around the anterior border of the diaphragmatic group to reach their undersurface, and decussate with the contralateral muscle behind the rectum and below the anterior sacrococcygeal ligament, blending anteriorly with the conjoined longitudinal muscle. This was puborectalis. Two further muscles arose from this line of origin from the pubis, the more anterior passing almost directly down, medially and back to insert into the posterolateral aspect of the apex of the prostate and membranous urethra, — the pubourethralis. Finally, arising behind pubourethralis, a distinct muscle bundle passed back, medially and down completing its course in an areolar tunnel to insert into the superolateral angle of the perineal body — the puboperineus. Muscle attachments of the lower layer extended more medially reaching the lower part of the symphysis to cross the inferolateral surface of the pubourethralis, puboperineus and puboanalis, and blend with the posterior third of the deep sphincter ani below the puboanalis sling, as part of puborectalis. In the female, puboanalis made up the whole of the superior layer at its attachment (Fig. 11).

Shafik (1975) believed puborectalis was part of the external anal sphincter and did not belong to levator ani. He made this statement since he could not differentiate the two, either morphologically or histologically, and described puborectalis as a U-shaped loop, the

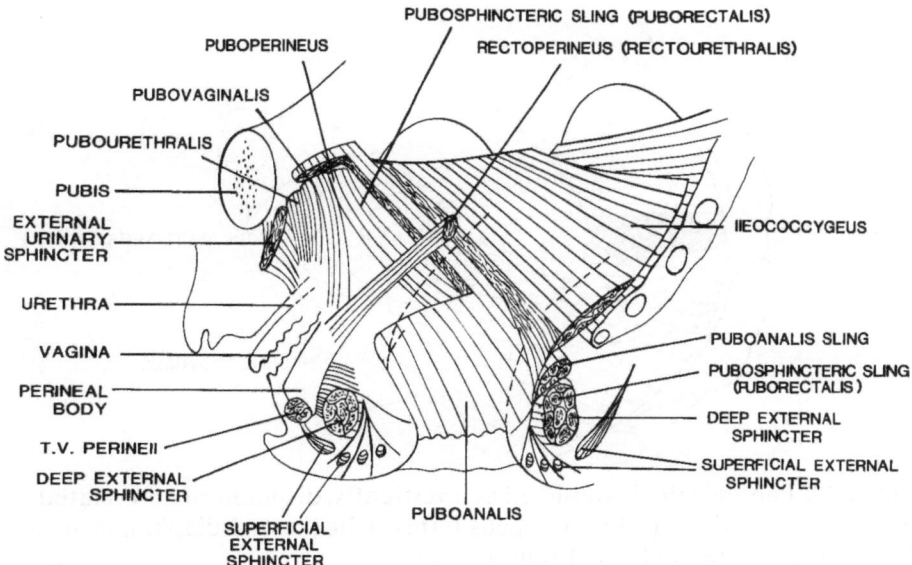

Figure 11. Muscles of the pelvic floor together with the urinary and anal sphincters in a female infant. The urethra, vagina and rectum are shown by dotted lines with the puboanalis partly cut away. (From Lawson)

two limbs of which formed a vertically lying ribbon closely related to the upper anal canal. The muscle bundles were fleshy, thicker and more condensed than those of levator, and tendinous fibres were not detected. Moreover a fibrous raphe did not exist posteriorly and it lay at a lower level than and under cover of the pubococcygeus, suggesting the two muscles were quite distinct anatomically (Fig. 12). Puborectalis sent a prolongation downward along the anal canal to join and share in the formation of the longitudinal anal muscle. Muscle bundles of both puborectalis and the deep external sphincter were found fused and could not be differentiated. The levator hiatus, he indicated, was formed by the medial borders of pubococcygeus, not puborectalis. A hiatal ligament of dense fascia bound intrahiatal viscera together, and to the edges of the hiatus (Fig. 13).

Ayoub (1978) studied the origin, direction, course and mode of termination of different groups of fibres originating in the anterior portion of levator ani which he dissected into three layers, termed pelvic, middle and perineal. The pelvic layer was a thin sheet of par-

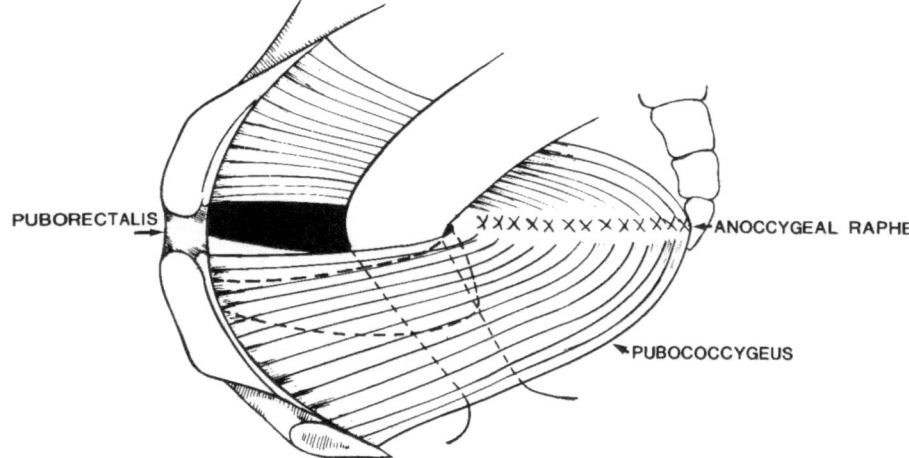

Figure 12. Puborectalis is depicted as a vertically disposed ribbon related to the anal canal whilst pubococcygeus forms a horizontal diaphragm which stretches across the pelvis. (From Shafik)

allel muscle bundles with a fleshy origin from the pelvic surface of the pubic body and anterior white lin :, the more anterior fibres coming into close contact with the side of the prostate to terminate by attachment to its capsule. In the female, the fibres ended by fusing with the outer coat of the lateral vaginal wall. The next group of fibres from this same layer formed a broader sheet which termi-

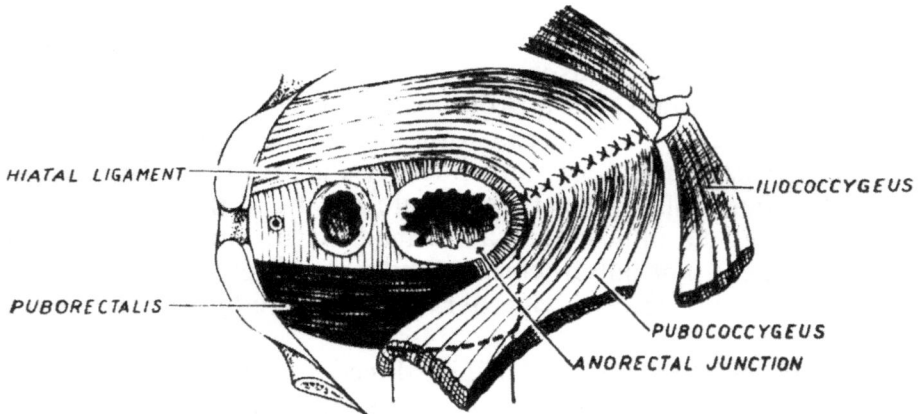

Figure 13. The hiatal ligament fills and packs the space between pubococcygeus and structures passing through the hiatus. (From Shafik)

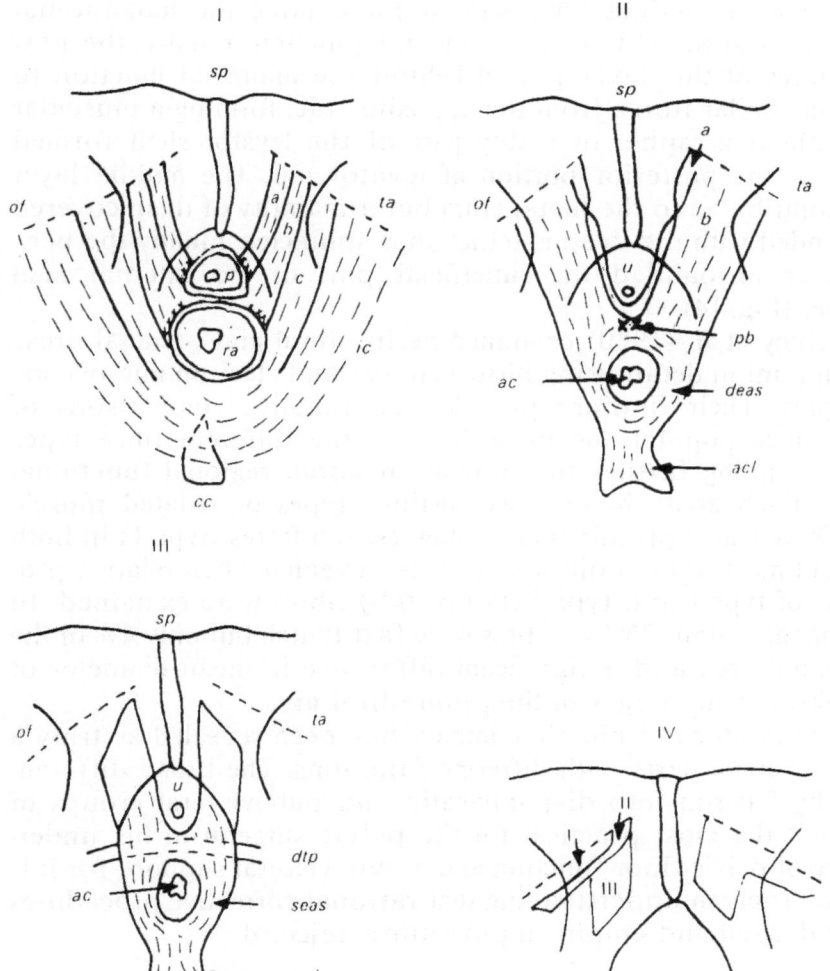

Figure 14. These 4 line drawings represent the 3 layers of the anterior fibres of the levator ani. i. Pelvic layer fibres a, b, c. ii. Middle layer fibres a, b. iii. Perineal layer fibres. iv. Origins of pelvic i, middle ii, and perineal iii fibre layers. *p* prostate; *ra* rectoanal junction; *c* coccyx; *ic* iliococcygeus; *pb* perineal body; *deas* deep external anal sphincter; *acl* anococcygeal ligament; *ac* anal canal; *u* urethra; *seas* superficial external anal sphincter; *dtp* deep transverse perinei. (From Ayoub)

nated by intermingling with and supplementing the longitudinal muscle layer at the side of the anorectal junction. Finally, the posterior fibres of this layer passed behind the anorectal junction to fuse with similar fibres from the opposite side, forming a muscular sling without a raphe, in reality part of the levator shelf formed mainly by the posterior portion of levator ani. The middle layer fibres contributed to the hiatal crura but a majority of them covered and blended with the deep external anal sphincter. Finally the perineal layer surrounded the superficial part of the external anal sphincter (Fig. 14).

Critchley et al. (1980) examined periurethral and perianal areas of levator ani in detail using histochemical and electron microscope techniques. Their findings provided quantitative comparisons of muscle fibre populations in each area, the different fibre types detected leading further to information about regional functional activity. Each area showed two distinct types of striated muscle fibre. There was a prominence of slow-twitch fibres (type 1) in both areas, but marked area differences were revealed when relative proportions of type 1 and type 2 (fast twitch) fibres were examined. In the perianal region, 23% of fibres were fast twitch but only 4% in the periurethral area and a significant difference in mean diameter of these fibres, being larger in the periurethral area.

So the levator ani muscle complex has been revealed as truly a muscle of many parts with differing functions. The broad differentiation by Lawson into diaphragmatic and pubovisceral groups of muscles is the most practical for the pelvic surgeon in his understanding of pelvic floor function and pelvic visceral support, for it is only with such an understanding that rational corrective procedures may be devised and empirical procedures rejected.

iii) Pouch of Douglas

In any consideration of the role of anatomic factors in the genesis of pulsion enterocoele, the anatomy of the pouch of Douglas must be explored fully. Important features are its boundaries and attachments to underlying tissues and the structures against which it rests, thus limiting its extension anteriorly, posteriorly, inferiorly, and laterally (Zacharin, 1980).

Posteriorly, the sac adheres intimately to the adventitial coat of the anterior and lateral aspects of the upper third of the rectum; it is reflected forward across the levator muscles and hiatus without adherence, to turn upward and become related to the upper third of the posterior vaginal wall. It has only a loose attachment to the vaginal wall, but as it ascends to the cervix the connection becomes closer. It cannot be stripped from either the cervix or upper rectal walls, yet between these attachments it can be mobilized completely and easily. Laterally, the peritoneal lining of this sac follows the contours of the lateral pelvic wall, riding freely over the great vessels, but gains a firm attachment to the ureter and subperitoneal tissues immediately inferior to the ureter. Therefore near the level of the true pelvic brim the sac adheres firmly to subperitoneal tissues, and apart from these corrective and stabilizing attachments it is very mobile. No doubt this mobility is associated with functions of rectal filling and vaginal movement. Although the rectovaginal septum is independent of both rectum and vagina, it tends to follow vaginal rather than rectal movement. There is great variability in its adequacy and completeness; all fibres run in a craniocaudal direction, arranged in two easily separable layers.

The cervix and upper vagina are suspended firmly in the pelvic cavity by the pelvic cellular tissues (Fig. 15) whereas the lower vagina is adherent densely to the margins of the levator crura and below that to the urogenital diaphragm which fills the space between the ischiopubic rami (Fig. 16 a, b). The urogenital diaphragm is composed of the deep and superficial perineal pouches and their contents and was developed to support midline structures when the ischiopubic symphysis became a pubic symphysis. It is less well developed in the female due to passage of the vagina, nevertheless it it exceedingly strong, since fractures of the rami commonly are compound into the vagina. The urogenital membrane (perineal membrane, triangular ligament) attaches to a bony ridge which runs forward along the ramus from the falciform crest posteriorly. Superiorly the deep pouch contains the compressor urethrae and deep transverse perineal muscle, and below, the superficial pouch holds the superficial transverse perineal muscle, the clitoral crura and the ischiocavernosus muscles. The levator crura attach to the vagina at the point where it enters the urogenital diaphragm, outlining a space filled with fat and limited by the lateral pelvic wall and urogenital diaphragm — the ischio-rectal fossa (Fig. 17).

Therefore, a characteristic feature of vaginal anatomy is the rel-

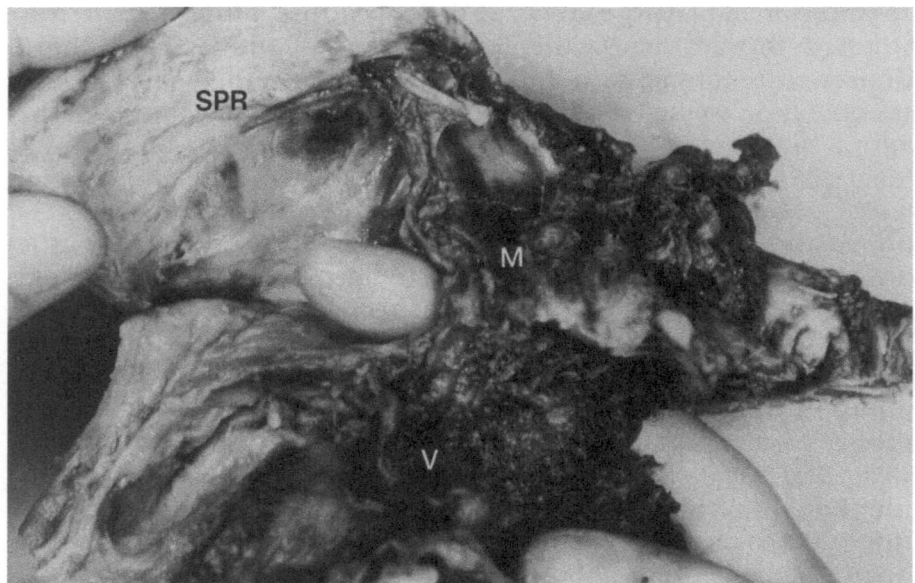

Figure 15. Pelvic view of the right anterior hemipelvis with the index finger passed beneath the pelvic cellular tissue bundle which is attached to the upper vagina and cervix. *M* Mackenrodt ligament; *V* upper vagina; *SPR* superior pubic ramus

ative fixation at the upper and lower ends, but it is mobile between these points. Upon division of the pelvic cellular tissue bundle (Mackenrodt), the vagina may be stripped easily to the margin of the levator hiatus. This step is employed during radical surgical removal of the vagina (Fig. 18). The levator complex is a most variable feature of pelvic floor anatomy. Morphologically, it is a bilateral group of muscles, with the exception of the puborectalis component, which is a single continuous muscle. Collectively, it is a broad thin muscle that arises anteriorly from the inner surface of the pubic bone lateral to the symphysis pubis and posteriorly from the base of the ischial spine. Between these two bony points, it takes origin from the obturator internus fascia, the so-called white line (Fig. 19). The puborectalis contribution lies most medially, arising from the inner surface of the pubic bones and outlining an apparent space centrally — the levator hiatus — through which the urethra, vagina and rectum pass from the pelvis to the perineum.

The main bulk of the muscle swings down and back to fuse and

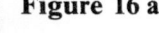

Figure 16 a

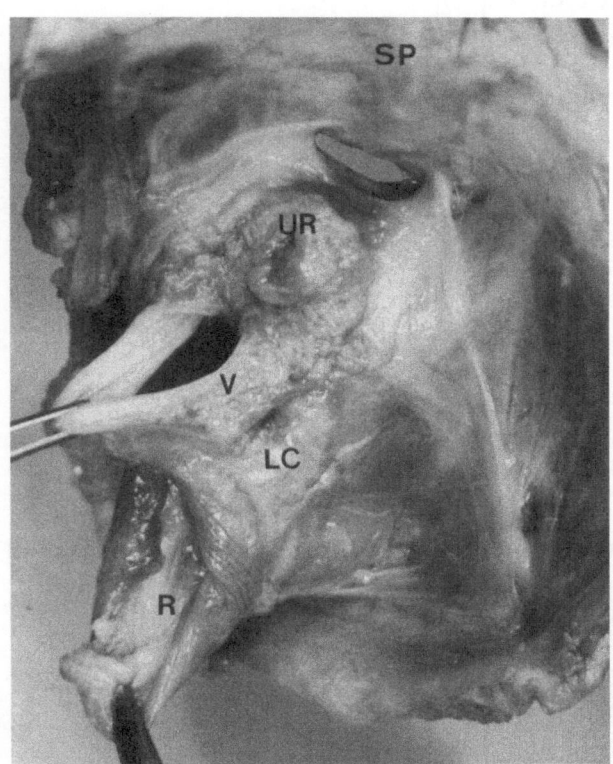

Figure 16 a, b. The dense fixation of the vagina to the margins of the levator crura are shown in these two photographs. *LC* levator crus; *UR* urethra; *B* bladder; *R* rectum; *SP* symphysis pubis; *V* vagina; *UT* ureter

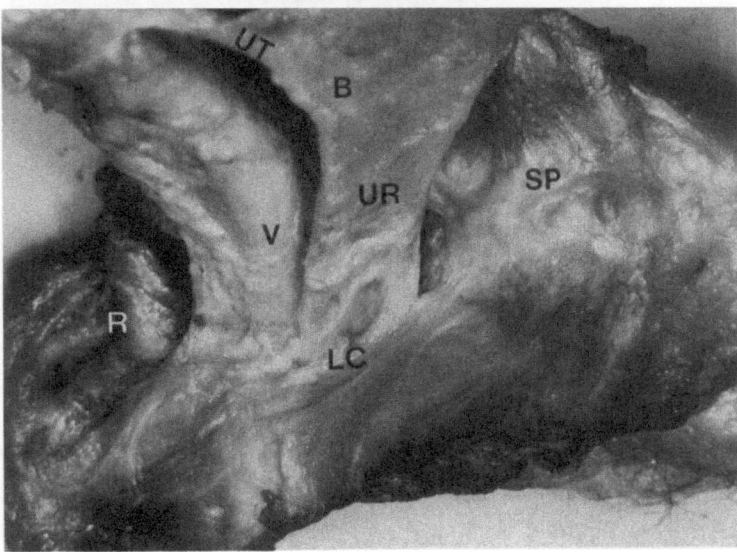

Figure 16 b

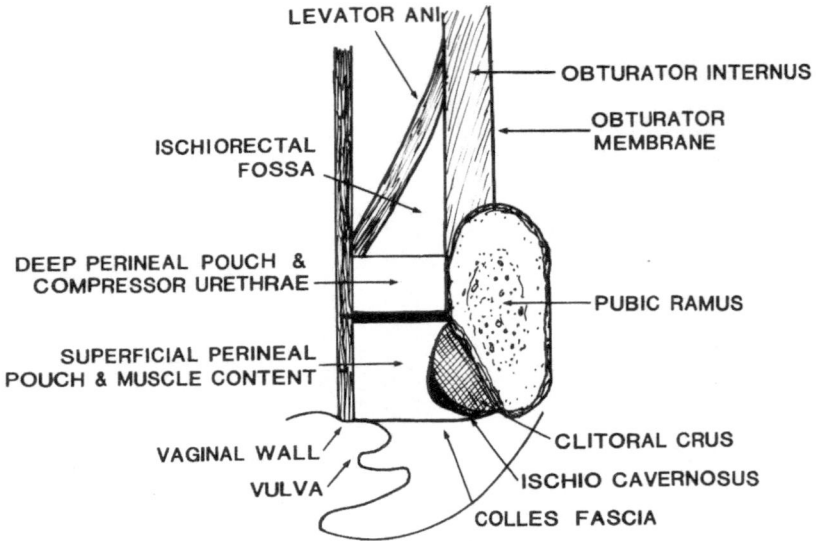

Figure 17. Diagram of the anatomical relationships at the urogenital diaphragm

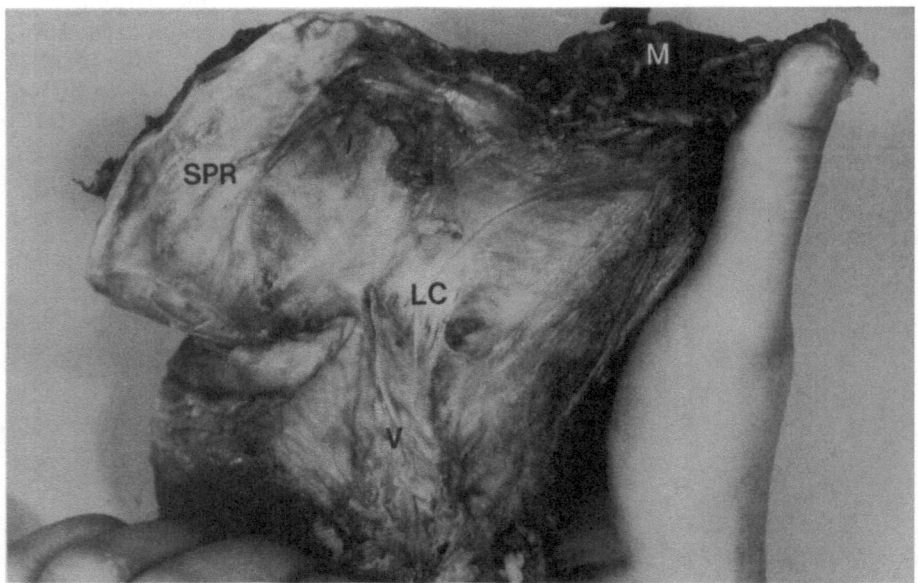

Figure 18. Right anterior hemipelvis showing the mobilisation of the vagina to the levator hiatus which is possible following division of the Mackenrodt tissue. *M* Mackenrodt tissue; *LC* levator crus; *V* vagina; *SPR* superior pubic ramus

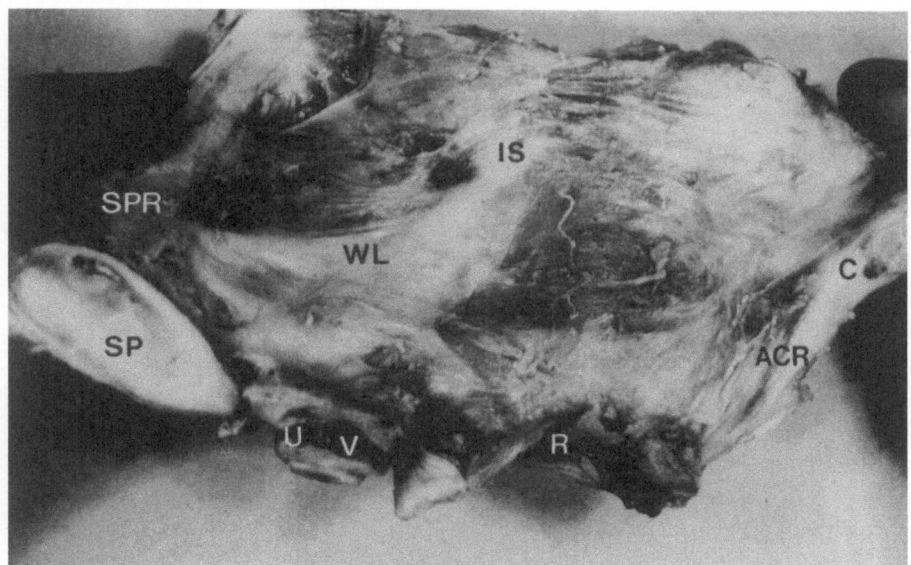

Figure 19. The right hemipelvis showing the levator complex, the white line origin and the structures traversing the levator hiatus.
SP symphysis pubis; *WL* white line; *C* coccyx; *V* vagina; *U* urethra; *SPR* superior pubic ramus; *IS* ischial spine; *ACR* anococcygeal raphe; *R* rectum

insert in a median raphe between the coccyx and the anal canal, the anococcygeal raphe or levator plate (Fig. 20 a, b). The puborectalis muscle takes no direct part in the formation of the plate, although it lies upon it enjoying a functional connection. The medial margins of the hiatus formed by puborectalis are termed the levator crura, and are attached firmly to both vagina and rectum. The crural relation to the urethra is more in the nature of a suburethral grooved platform without direct attachment, as compared with the other two structures. Posteriorly, below the peritoneal reflection, the rectum is exceedingly mobile above the levator complex, whereas laterally the pelvic wall, obturator muscles, and levator origin normally control the shape of the pouch of Douglas. The major variable in the normal levator complex is the quality of muscle development. Usually, the margin of the hiatus and the levator plate contain thick muscle bundles, but with progress laterally toward the obturator fascia, the muscle tissue usually diminishes in thickness quite obviously, so that when the "white line" area is reached, only a thin

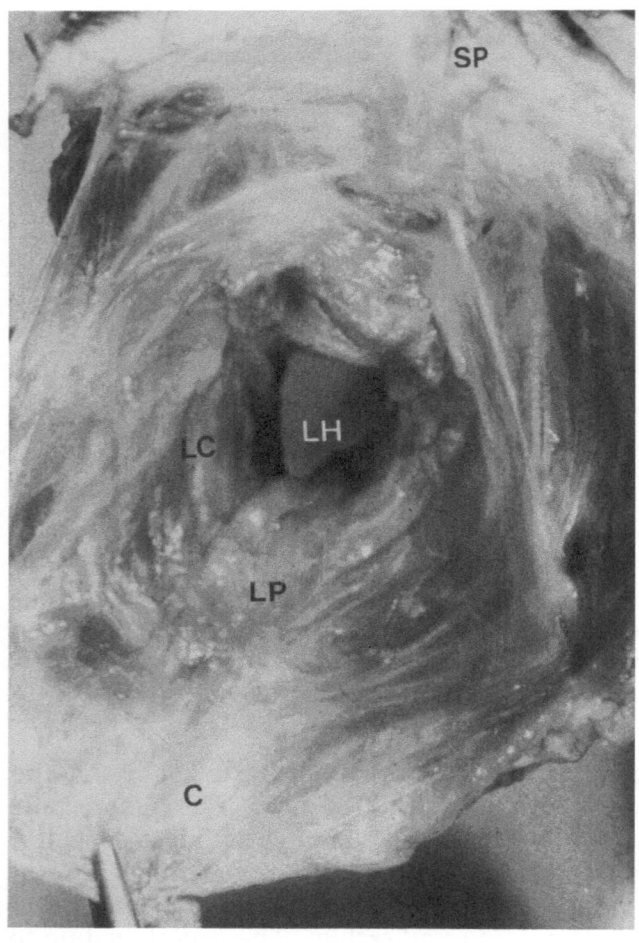

Figure 20 a

Figure 20 a, b. The levator complex viewed from above (**a**) and a close up of the levator plate area (**b**). *SP* symphysis pubis; *LC* levator crus; *C* coccyx; *LH* levator hiatus; *LP* levator plate

membrane devoid of muscle tissue remains. This general description of muscle loss laterally is accentuated particularly in obese women and in women of advancing age. There is also a correlation of levator muscle mass to general body musculature.

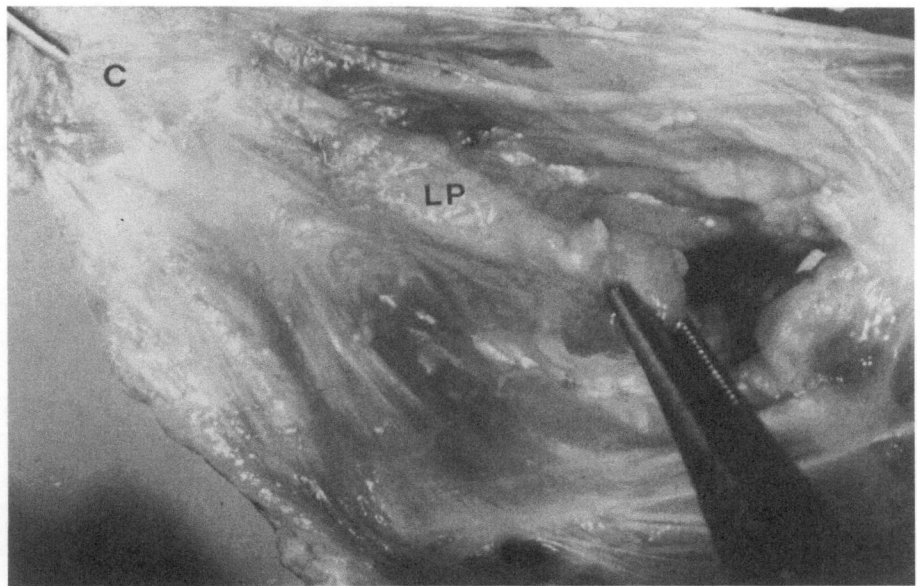

Figure 20 b

Comparative Anatomy

i) Human

It is well known that mechanical problems affecting the pelvic floor in the human female — genital prolapse including enterocoele, and stress incontinence of urine — are very uncommon in certain racial groups e.g. Chinese, Eskimo, African and American Negro. If this is indeed so, dissection of the pelvic floor should demonstrate important anatomical differences between Oriental and Occidental females. An anatomical study of 30 Chinese females ranging in age from 12 to 83 years (Zacharin, 1977) was made to elucidate differences. Particular features noted in each subject were the configuration of the bony pelvis, the anatomy of the pouch of Douglas and general macroscopic appearances of the levator complex. Removal of a large part of the anterior pelvis enabled a detailed examination

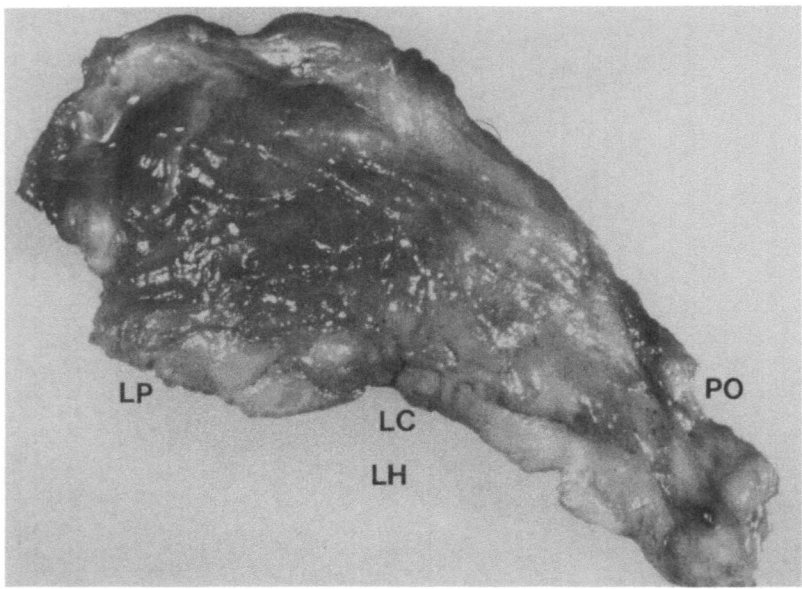

Figure 21. The left half of the levator complex in a young Chinese female showing the exceedingly thick muscle tissue with minimal aponeurosis. *PO* pubic origin; *LP* levator plate; *LC* levator crus; *LH* levator hiatus

of the muscle to be made, and overall a consistent pattern was observed. The levator complex could be seen clearly, and on either side the muscle mass was elevated from the ischiorectal fossa to judge thickness and general quality. Measurements of levator plate length and crural thickness were made, and several muscles examined microscopically. In 24 of 30 women, the whole complex, crura and plate were described as normal, but in 14, the tissues were considered much better developed than in Occidental females, in that the muscle was thicker and fibres extended further laterally toward the "white line" origin than in the Occidental. The plate and crural areas were particularly thickened — extremely so in certain subjects — and connective tissue binding anal canal, vagina and urethra to the crural margins was notably strong and dense (Fig. 21). Most subjects had very well developed pelvic cellular tissues. This assessment was made on thickness and general texture of the param- etrium following its isolation by opening the paravesical and para- rectal spaces widely.

Although general anatomical details of the pouch of Douglas

resembled those of the Occidental female, nevertheless there were noteworthy differences in a third of the subjects examined. Standard anatomy describes the upper third of the vagina covered by peritoneum, but in 10 females the peritoneum covered nearly two-thirds of the vagina, forming a particularly deep pouch. Associated with this excessively deep pouch was a remarkable degree of genital tract and rectal mobility, which would certainly permit easy movement of the genital tract over the levator plate in response to a sudden increase in intra-abdominal pressure, yet at the same time, limitation of descent because of stronger parametrial tissues could compensate for this increased mobility.

In 27 Chinese subjects the relationship of the levator complex to the urethra although similar, was qualitatively and quantitatively different from the Occidental pattern. The muscle mass in most was

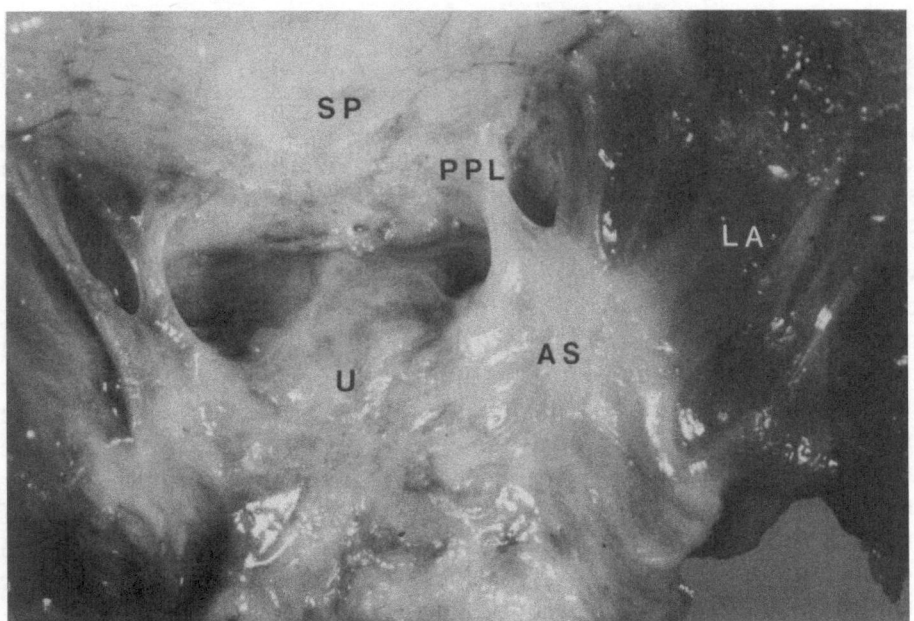

Figure 22. Pelvic surface of the pubic symphysis in a young Chinese female, viewed from above. The well-developed levator muscle on either side is seen, relatively deficient posterior pubourethral ligaments and the exceedingly dense aponeurotic sheet extending between the levator muscles and supporting the urethra. *SP* symphysis pubis; *PPL* posterior pubourethral ligament; *AS* aponeurotic sheet; *LA* levator ani; *U* urethra

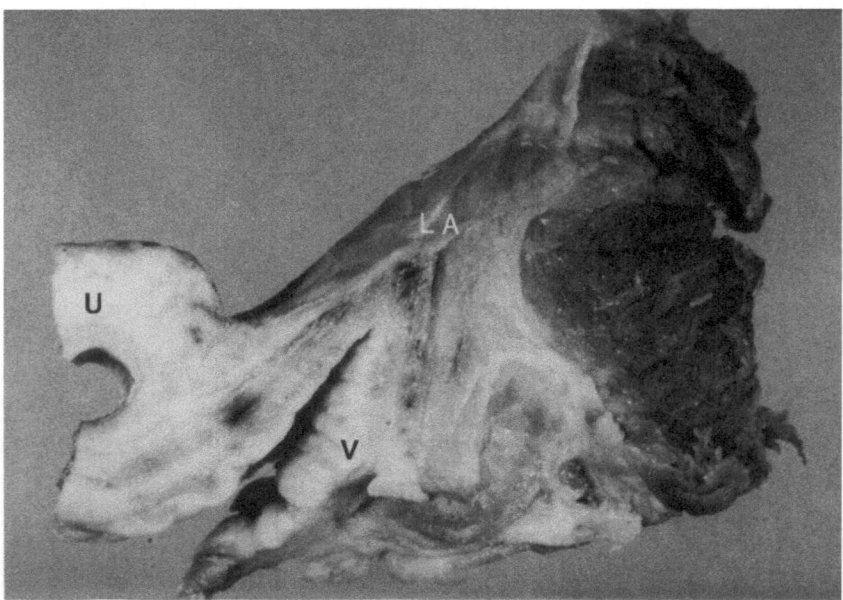

Figure 23. Coronal section through the urethra in a young Chinese female, at the junction of the upper ⅓ and lower ⅔. The method of urethral suspension by musculo-aponeurotic sling from the lateral pelvic wall is demonstrated clearly. *U* urethra; *V* vagina; *LA* levator ani

well or very well developed and the pelvic surface was covered by a dense fascial sheet, so thick in some as to hide the underlying muscle bundles. As it approached the urethra it thickened noticeably, particularly at the point where the posterior pubo-urethral ligament fused with it. This fascial sheet decussated in the midline with its fellow and fused strongly with the fascia of the urethral roof. The urethra was seen to be suspended from the levator muscle by this fascial extension, the thickness and toughness of muscle and fascia providing such undoubted strength and resilience for the urethral suspensory mechanism, that support by posterior ligaments seemed almost redundant.

In the Chinese, the urethra is therefore powerfully and elastically suspended as though upon a trampoline, to rise and fall with changes in intra-abdominal pressure (Fig. 22, 23) and these findings enabled the following conclusions to be reached. Probably, tissue quality is the real reason why low socio-economic status Chinese women develop genital prolapse and enterocoele rarely, and urinary stress incontinence almost never. Nor does the commonly found deep pouch of Douglas predispose to enterocoele. The reasons for such anatomy must include a genetic influence, generations of hard work, and a diet which makes obesity uncommon; but perhaps the major factor contributing to levator and pelvic cellular tissue excellence is the squatting position adopted for resting, childbirth and defaecation. In the Westernised Chinese female, it is known that genital prolapse occurs in such women but still is of lesser incidence than the Occidental females. One could theorise perhaps that the changed incidence might well be related to deterioration in pelvic anatomy and function as a consequence of accepting Western habits. It seems that the incidence of prolapse does not begin to change until several generations have been exposed to Western influences with an increasing departure from their ethnic way of life.

ii) *Ruminant Animals*

Ruminant farm animals, particularly the cow and ewe are prone to genital prolapse. Occasionally the mare, bitch and sow are affected, and the fact that prolapse occurs at all in four-footed animals, is reason for interest and further investigation since apparently their antigravity position does not protect them. There is a worldwide incidence in the ewe, the frequency depending upon the breed of sheep, and husbandry methods employed. Greatest numbers occur in mature sheep, developing in late gestation, and increasing with successive pregnancies. Occasionally prolapse follows delivery and rarely the condition may occur apart from pregnancy. In early cases, prolapse occurs only when the animal lies down; but later protrusion is evident when standing progressing to total eversion (Fig. 24 a). When spontaneous reduction no longer occurs, the skin dries and becomes grossly infected. Amongst cattle, beef breeds such as Herefords are affected mainly.

The theories of aetiology advanced by veterinarians include poor quality feed and vitamin D deficiency, the latter also being blamed for umbilical and inguinal herniae. Since special breeds are more prone and hereditary predisposition has been suggested, offenders usually are culled and prevented from further breeding. Vaginal eversion has been thought due to the increased thickening of vaginal

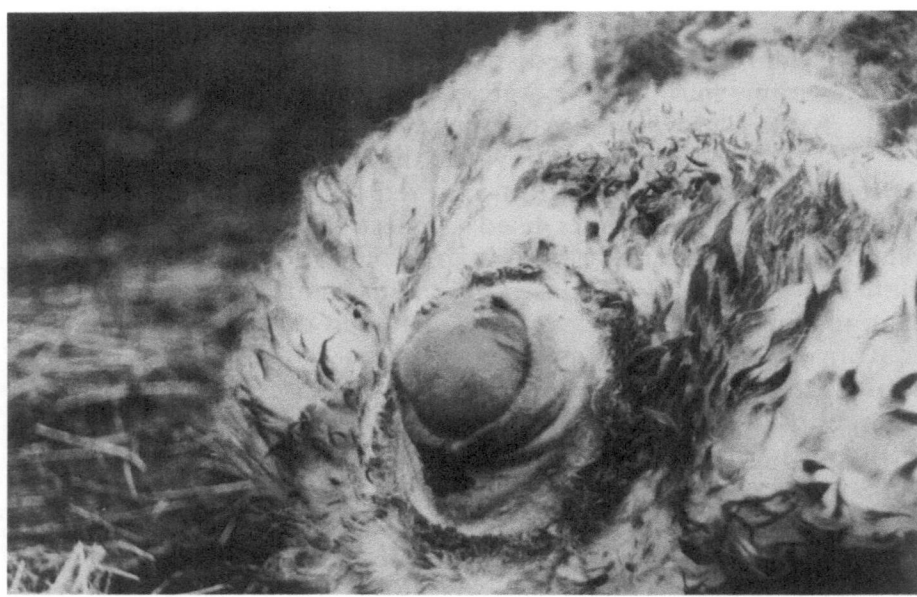

Figure 24 a. A well developed genital prolapse in a pregnant ewe evident in the standing position

epithelium resulting from a high oestrogen intake, and may also predispose to straining which is accentuated when the prolapse has commenced. Prolapse is much more common in sheep on hilly country, for they tend to lie with their buttocks directed downhill and pregnant ewes commonly develop prolapse in the downhill position since field studies have shown mud on the cervix. Investigations which helped elucidate the aetiology of this condition in the ewe, were conducted at Lincoln College, Christchurch, New Zealand (McLean and Claxton, 1960). Measurements of intra-abdominal pressure and pelvic laxity were taken during pregnancy from within the peritoneal cavity, on the abdominal wall and within the vagina, and readings were taken with the animal standing and lying, and also with the buttocks directed down a slope of 16°. Fluctuations due to respiration, change of stance etc., were minimised by waiting five minutes before taking readings.

Pressure at the pelvic inlet while standing was negative; but positive when lying and increased greatly in the "buttocks downhill" position, the range being −5 cms to +30 cms of water. Weight increase in the ewe due to diet and/or pregnancy, could cause a rise of up to 30 cms of water, higher again when the downhill position was assumed, but pressure rises due to pregnancy or overeating could be compensated partly by abdominal wall stretch. These findings strongly suggested that marked intra-abdominal pressure rise occurred with pregnancy, overeating and the downhill position. Respiratory embarrassment was the factor which caused cessation of feeding, relieved by assumption of the downhill position. Pelvic inlet pressure was increased further by straining to relieve an over-full bladder. It seemed these factors produced a critical pressure, not compensated fully by abdominal wall stretch, so pressure release was sought through the pelvic canal but the ewes were able to resist this pressure increase without developing vaginal eversion because of laxity of the pelvic structures.

Measurements of vaginal and vulval distensibility during pregnancy, showed a marked increase with return to normal values approximately two weeks after lambing. Loosening of pelvic joints could be demonstrated radiologically and by dissection, and ewes with a previous prolapse showed higher readings of pelvic laxity measurements at an earlier stage in pregnancy than normal.

Results of pelvic dissection in the cow and ewe (Zacharin, 1969) showed the following features — in both, the distal vagina and vulva were supported flexibly at the pelvic outlet by a series of fascial sheets similar to the human perineal membrane. The vulva was surrounded by constrictor vulvae and vestibular muscles with connections to retractor ani, sphincter ani and the suspensory ligament of the anus. Levator ani was the tail mover, and its origin did not extend onto the pubis.

Veterinary texts indicate faith in the support value of the broad ligament yet dissection showed it flimsy and without any condensation of retroperitoneal cellular tissues equivalent to the human (Fig. 24 b). Nevertheless in principle, the mechanical set-up was similar to the human, since there was no direct support between firm vulvovaginal attachments inferiorly, and the less strong attachments at the level of entry of the uterine vessels above, even though the upper attachments mechanically were worthless. Probably the pelvic relaxation of pregnancy associated with the pregnant uterus, over-feeding, a downhill lie, and an accentuated vaginal eversion due to straining, would be enough to produce prolapse in the ewe. The major difference in genital tract anchorage between the human female and ruminant animals occurs in the upper tract where dense

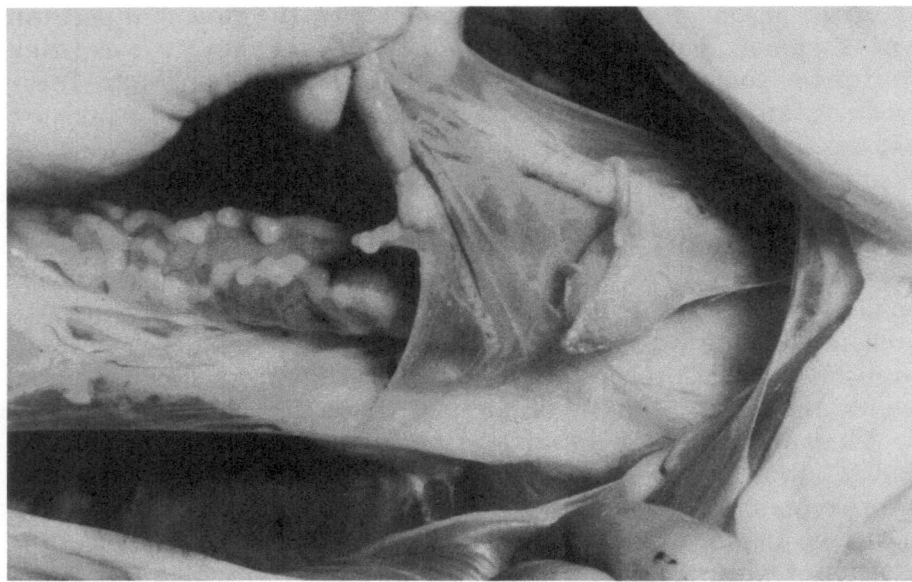

Figure 24 b. Traction applied to the uterus of a ewe demonstrating the flimsy transparent nature of the broad ligament

pelvic cellular connective tissue thickening related to the vascular pedicle in the human is lacking entirely in the animal, but its absence possibly is compensated by the four-footed position, which whilst not conferring immunity, certainly seems important in the cure that follows delivery. There have been many reports of vaginal and uterine prolapse in animals — sheep, buffalo, dairy cows, pigmy hippopotamus, siamese cat, donkey mare and sow. Pregnancy is the common factor and the management was entirely symptomatic.

Functional Anatomy

Dickinson (1869) commented that the "fleshy diaphragm called the pelvic floor had a peculiar function, in that it must close up and completely seal the lower end of the body cavity, resisting strong and frequent pressure, it must open up and leave completely free the lower end of the cavity, must make away with itself when occasion demands, and yet resume its other function with unimpaired integrity". Professor Berry Hart had divided the pelvic floor into two segments which he termed pubic and sacral, the pubic segment consisting of loose tissue — bladder, urethra, anterior vaginal wall etc., and attached anteriorly to the pubic symphysis. The sacral segment joined to the coccyx and sacrum and comprised rectum and perineum, together with tendinous and muscular tissue (Fig. 25). During labour both segments could be likened to folding doors, for uterine action pulled up the pubic, and drove the child against the sacral. This action was analogous to the way one passed through two folding doors, pulling one door forward and pushing the other away. Dickinson believed the pelvic floor was constructed similarly to the inguinal canal, in two layers with an opening in each. The thick pubic segment or upper layer, had a thin circle of attachment to the sacrum, through which a cleft — the inner aperture — opened between the uterosacral ligaments (Fig. 26). A canal, the vagina, ran

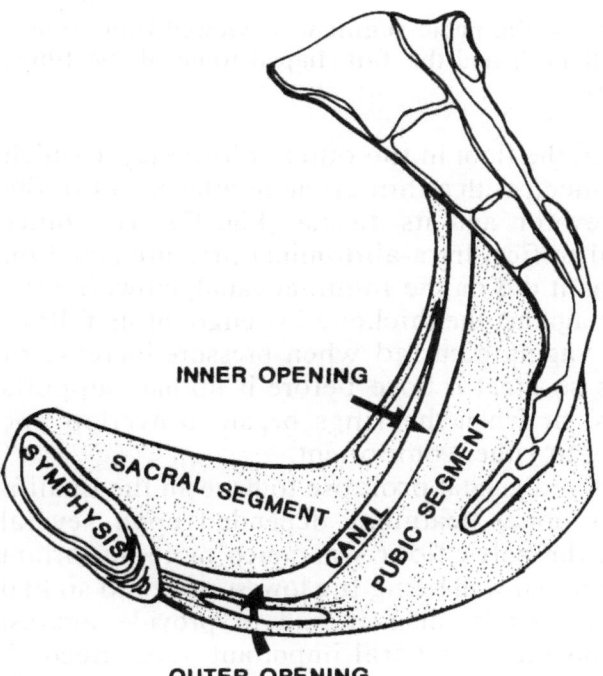

Figure 25. The pubic and sacral segments with their attachments according to Berry Hart, showing the resemblance to the inguinal canal

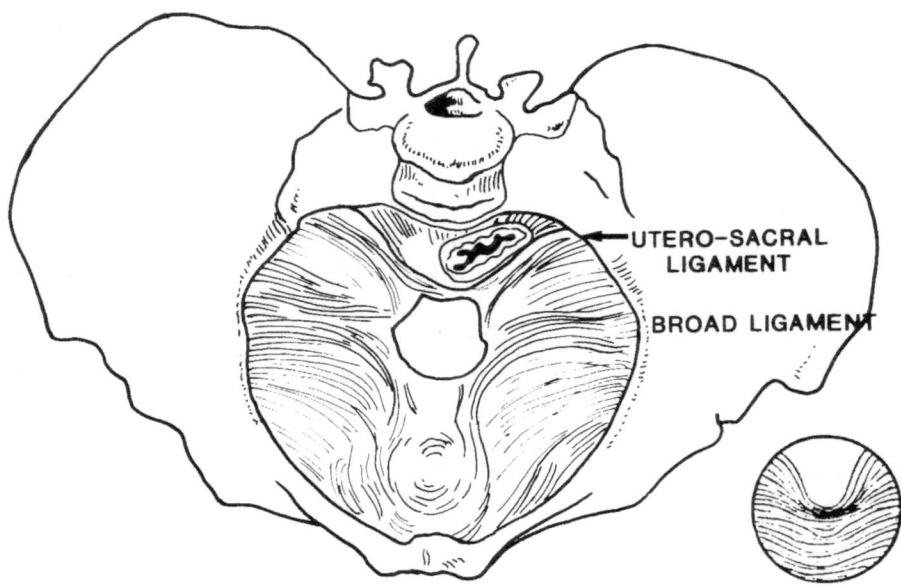

UTERO-SACRAL
LIGAMENT

BROAD LIGAMENT

Figure 26. The upper layer — the pubic segment — viewed from above. The inner aperture is well back and the fan-shaped trend of the fibres depicted. (From Dickinson)

obliquely down from it to the floor in the outer or lower layer which was the thick sacral segment, with a thin circle of attachment to the pubic bones, mainly levator and its fascia (Fig. 27). The outer opening was the vaginal orifice. Intra-abdominal pressure acted on the closed pelvic floor as it did on the inguinal canal, crowding the weak part of each layer against the thickened strength of its fellow. Prolapse of uterus and vagina occurred when pressure increase or weight from above was so great it bore before it normal supports made up of two layers, or when the rings began to overlap one another following injury to either component.

Barrett (1909) considered genital prolapse to have all the qualifications of hernia, so rational treatment depended upon several important points. First, the pelvic floor was much more important than the rest of the abdominal wall being the lowest part, and so had to withstand the greatest strain, also it had to provide against "faults" caused by the passage of several important tracts. Second, the pelvic floor had much greater importance in the human female than in the mammal where the longitudinal axis of the body was horizontal, so little weight fell on the perineum.

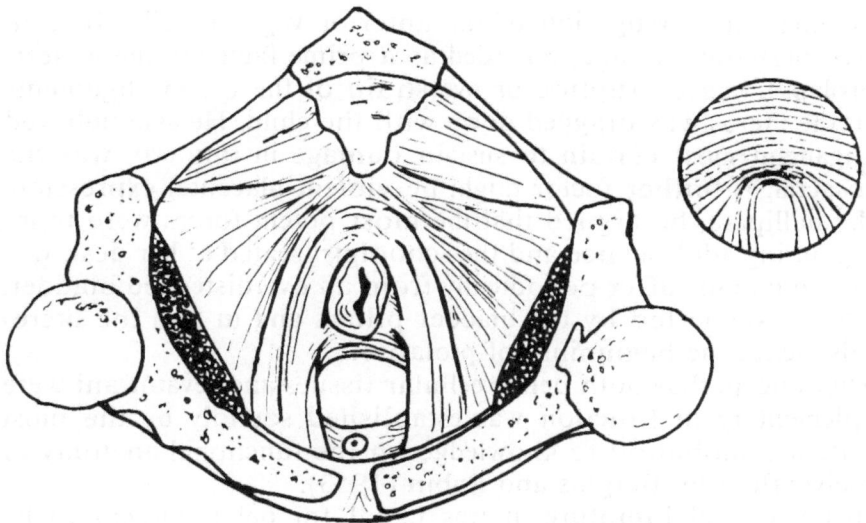

Figure 27. The under layer — the sacral segment — seen from above. The opening is situated well forward and the fan-shape of the fibres is opposite in direction to those shown in Fig. 26. (From Dickinson)

Sturmdorf (1919) summarised the function of the levator concisely, stating that it diminished the force of intra-abdominal pressure upon the pelvic contents by deflecting its direction, and augmented resistance to it by closing the uterovaginal angle so obstructing the pelvic outlet by compressing the vaginal canal. Also it was a tensor of the pelvic fascia, the antagonist of the diaphragm and abdominal muscles, and when intact maintained the equilibrium of the pelvic organs.

Thelander (1922) believed the cardinal ligaments were all important and acted in opposition to intra-abdominal pressure, steadying the uterus in its normal position. To do this adequately they had to be very powerful, for the resultant upward pull of two almost horizontal ligaments was small. Therefore, providing they remained intact, their upward pull increased with uterine descent as the angle at which they acted became less obtuse. The resultant force exerted by the uterosacrals, was directly in the line of the vaginal canal so tension of these bands would cause tension to the longitudinal bands of the anterior vaginal wall — the pillars of the bladder — and relaxation of uterosacrals would be associated with shortening and corrugation of the anterior vaginal wall. He considered obstetric damage, regarded as a prime factor in the genesis of prolapse, caused rupture or overstrain of the uterine ligaments when the uterus was dragged down with the child. He also believed the ligament most certain to sustain damage in this way was the uterosacral. A further factor might be violent placental expression. In the nullipara, he argued that the most potent forces were those acting during adolescence and the schoolgirl seated at her desk was almost certain to suffer periodically from an overdistended bladder, which was supported by the bladder pillars and in turn the uterosacrals, hence the beginnings of prolapse.

The concept that both pelvic cellular tissues and levator ani were complementary in function was established soundly by the most important contribution to knowledge on the functional anatomy of the pelvic floor by Berglas and Rubin (1953).

In anatomical literature, it was usual for pelvic viscera to be shown situated over the pelvic aperture, and whilst true in the cadaver suggesting a funnel-shaped configuration of the pelvic diaphragm, also it was accepted as true for the living female (Fig. 28). Earlier authors who had described and explained levator function, focussed attention on hiatal closure effected by pubococcygeus and puborectalis for when these muscles contracted, it was believed they shortened lengthwise, gaining thickness and diminishing the pelvic floor aperture transversely, so reducing the anteroposterior diameter considerably. Simultaneously, the visceral canals were compressed from behind forward leading to their occlusion — the so-called H-shaped slit assumed by the vagina.

Whilst some narrowing of the hiatus due to muscle contraction could be observed in the living female, it was but a minor manifestation of the physiological action of the levator ani muscle, and the generally accepted description of pelvic viscera poised over the aperture in the pelvic diaphragm was not applicable to a living female with an intact pelvic floor. Levator myography in living females at rest, showed the levator plate was almost horizontal, with the uterus and vagina overlying it and not the hiatus. The cervix lay on the posterior part of the plate near to its insertion into the coccyx, separated from the plate by the posterior vaginal wall and rectum (Fig. 29). The vagina lay within the pelvis almost parallel to the plate, similar to the course of the terminal rectum and when the rectum filled, the uterus and vagina were forced forward, yet the

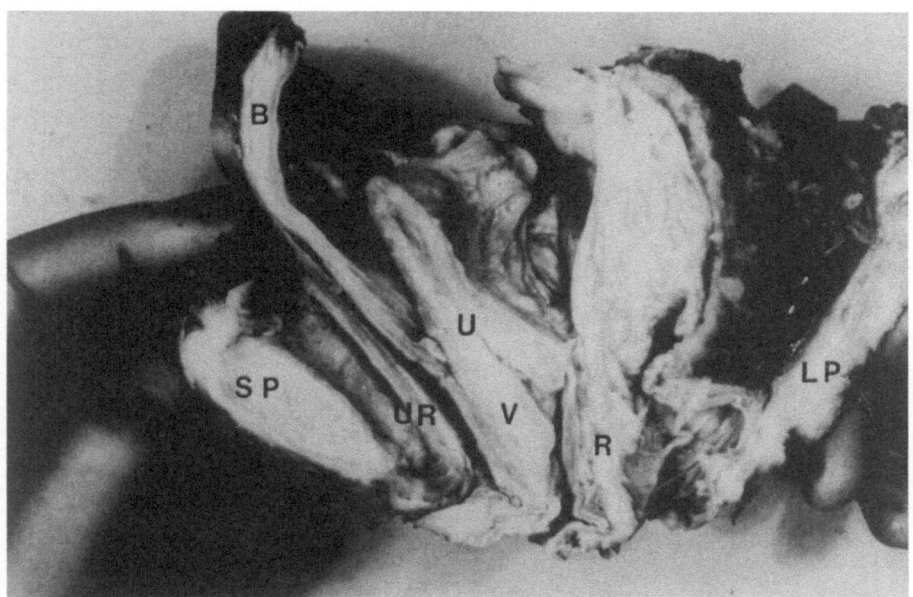

Figure 28. A usual anatomical photograph of the pelvic viscera poised over the pelvic outlet. *SP* symphysis pubis; *U* uterus; *V* vagina; *LP* levator plate; *B* bladder; *UR* urethra; *R* rectum

axis of the uterus remained poised over the plate. During straining, pressure in the abdominopelvic cavity rose as an effect of abdominal wall contraction and simultaneous contraction of the pelvic diaphragm. Since the diaphragm was fixed at both ends, resistance to shortening during contraction resulted in increased tension, with greater resistance to abdominopelvic pressure. Myography during straining, showed insignificant shortening of the longitudinal and transverse diameters of the hiatus, with a degree of occlusion incapable of preventing pelvic organ protrusion. The visceral thrust from above was directed backward and downward, pushing the uterus, vagina and rectum towards and against the plate, far behind the hiatus. So with an intact pelvic diaphragm, the pelvic floor aperture was out of reach of the effect of intra-abdominal pressure on the uterus. A retroverted uterus was treated in exactly the same way.

Adequate contraction of the levator plate capable of resisting downward thrust exerted by rising intra-abdominal pressure, presupposed all the attachments of the levator muscle were unim-

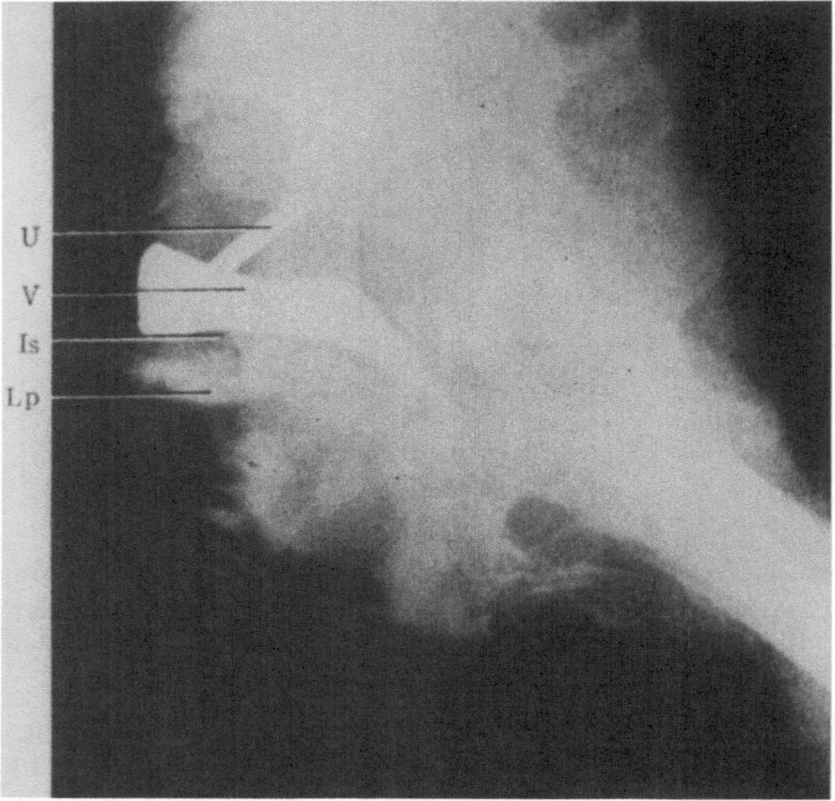

Figure 29. Lateral view of a 25 year old female recumbent and at rest. The levator plate is shown clearly with the vaginal long axis horizontal and parallel to the plate, contrary to the anatomy of Figure 28. Normally the vagina and uterus lie over the plate, not the hiatus. *U* uterus; *IS* ischial spine; *V* vagina; *LP* levator plate. (From Berglas and Rubin)

paired. When structural or functional integrity of the levator muscle was impaired, the plate correspondingly lost its capacity to contract adequately, lowering its power of resistance to increased intra-abdominal pressure, and so an altered relationship to the uterus occurred creating conditions predisposing to prolapse (Fig. 30 a, b). Following birth injury, lacerations of pubococcygeus and puborectalis have been described repeatedly, occurring usually in the muscle origin from the pubic bones, and involving the crura. Crural damage

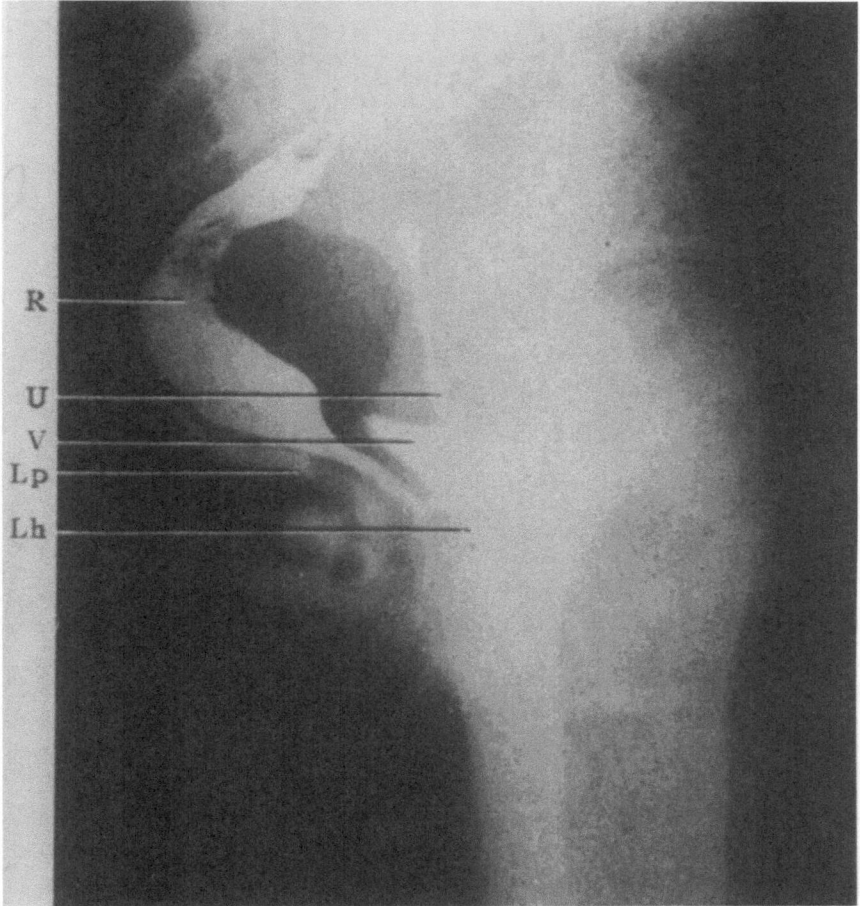

Figure 30 a. Lateral view of a nulliparous female with the clinical diagnosis of a relaxed pelvic floor. Although the plate is horizontal, the vagina and uterus lie over the hiatus, not the plate

led to changes in position of the levator plate within the pelvic outlet, with a loss of resilience and a tendency to sag. There was definite correlation between plate inclination and the degree of prolapse. When levator integrity was impaired, the greater inclination of the plate meant a smaller area of uterus overlying it and a larger portion of uterus over the hiatus. The degree of plate inclination determined both the length of the pelvic floor aperture and the resistance which the plate could exert against the thrust of intra-

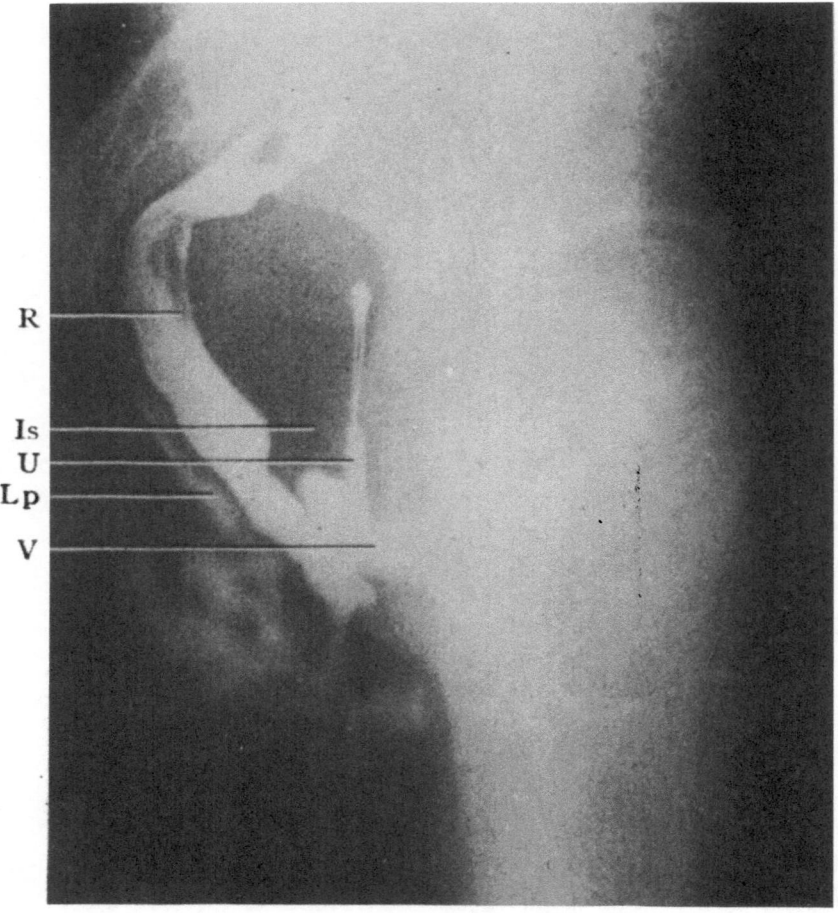

R

Is
U
Lp

V

Figure 30 b. Straining would increase plate inclination and the cervix and vagina would commence descent into the hiatus. (From Berglas and Rubin)

abdominal pressure. It was upon these two features that the degree of uterine descent depended. In first degree prolapse the plate at rest had a horizontal course, but even at rest the uterus failed to occupy its normal position over the posterior part of the plate. In second degree prolapse the plate at rest showed considerable inclination, the uterus being situated over the enlarged pelvic floor aperture, and in third degree prolapse, the plate was vertical, failing to give any support whatever to the uterus.

So the big step forward in appreciation of pelvic floor function came with this work, for it differed from all earlier investigations in two fundamental respects. Decisions were reached by considering the anatomy of living females, and the proper view was advanced that ascribing function to cadaveric anatomy not only was incorrect, it led to false conclusions.

Lawson (1974) said more specific things about levator ani function. The posterior group of obturator muscles performed a simple diaphragmatic role, whereas the anterior group, the pubovisceral muscles not only supported the viscera, but could by active contraction, draw the viscera upward and forward. Pubourethralis, vaginalis and analis, by nature of their insertion, also tended to draw the urethra, vagina and upper canal open, and could contribute to the rapid fall in pressure in the upper anal canal and urethra at the commencement of defaecation, and upon the initiation of micturition. On the other hand the sling fibres of the puboanalis, puborectalis and puboperineus acting through the perineal body, in addition to drawing up the viscera, would tend also to close off the urethra, vagina and anal canal.

Shafik (1975) suggested the levators contracted as a single sheet, reinforced at their central and most curved part by the anococcygeal raphe, which served also to prevent constrictive action by the levators on the intrahiatal contents. He believed the main brunt of intra-abdominal pressure fell upon the raphe and not the hiatus, since the former was more dependent. Increases could be opposed to a point at which the raphe was maximally shortened and broadened, then any increase beyond this limit would tend to throw the load onto the raphe and hiatus together, so the tendinous fibres could be stretched, and once stretched, they would not return to normal allowing the diaphragm to sag and the hiatus to widen with stretching of the hiatal ligament. Shafik considered that the puborectalis acted as a constrictor of the anorectal junction, contrasting with the levator which was a dilator (Fig. 31).

Ayoub (1978) considered the possible role of the levator muscle, particularly its anterior fibres, could well be fixation and prevention of prolapse of pelvic viscera which passed through the hiatus. Fibres of the middle and perineal layers could play an important role in anal canal fixation by providing a stable base for the external anal sphincter. Generally, however, the anterior fibres of the levator could be regarded as the visceral part of the muscle, and the pos-

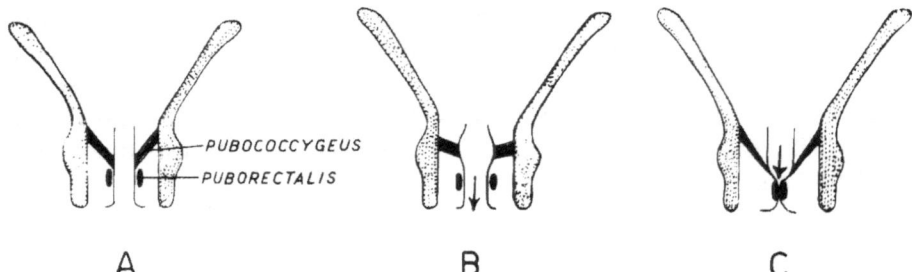

PUBOCOCCYGEUS
PUBORECTALIS

A   B   C

Figure 31 A—C. The mechanism of action of pubococcygeus and puborectalis.
A At rest; **B** During defaecation. Pubococcygeus contracts, elevates and widens the hiatus and then the pull upon the intrahiatal ligament widens the anorectal junction to produce evacuation. During this function, puborectalis is relaxed., **C** Opposition to the call to stool with puborectalis contracted and pubococcygeus relaxed. (From Shafik)

terior fibres the parietal part. He explained the relative thickness of the anterior fibres by the fact that they bore the weight of weight-bearing pelvic organs not supported by the bony pelvic walls.

Critchley et al. (1980) discussing the functional implications of their work on muscle fibre populations of levator ani, concluded that the muscle could not be considered as a single morphological or functional unit, since its constituent parts performed differing functions according to their anatomical locations, and of course the results they obtained regarding fibre populations, must be of considerable importance in the interpretation of myographic recordings obtained from single sites in the levator ani muscle. The predominance of type 1 fibres in both periurethral and perianal regions indicated the muscle was suited ideally to the maintenance of tone over long periods. The presence of a greater proportion of fast twitch fibres in the perianal region of the levator might correlate with the physiological characteristics of the constituent fibres of the external anal sphincter, for it was noteworthy that the perianal levator ani was in direct structural continuity with the external anal sphincter. Furthermore, component fibres of the external anal sphincter had similar histochemical properties to those of the perianal levator ani, whilst in contrast, the periurethral part of the levator consisted almost entirely of slow twitch fibres, anatomically separate from those which constituted the external urethral sphincter. The small proportion of relatively large diameter fast twitch fibres present in this part of the levator might be important in producing forces which caused sudden occlusion of the urethral lumen during coughing and sneezing. Collectively the results of their study showed the levator ani muscle could not be considered as a single morphological or functional unit.

Conclusions

Variations in intra-abdominal pressure must be balanced by adequate visceral support if herniation through the pelvic outlet is to be prevented. In the quadruped, shown by experimental evidence in the sheep, normally there is a negative intra-abdominal pressure at the pelvic inlet due no doubt to visceral weight falling forward and relying on the abdominal wall for support. The rise in intra-abdominal pressure produced by overeating leads to respiratory embarrassment largely compensated by the adoption of a downhill lying position. Critical change in the balance of forces comes with the softening of pregnancy, when intra-abdominal pressure exceeds pelvic floor resistance, and prolapse of the genital tract may result.

With the change from plantigrade to erect attitude, the pelvis and vertebral column of man underwent various evolutionary changes which restored balance between intra-abdominal pressure and visceral support, for clearly the method of visceral support in man needed to be more complex than that of fourfooted animals and was achieved by a combination of anatomical changes. The lumbosacral curve, a specific human characteristic, directed the viscera forward onto the abdominal wall and flattened pubic bones, so much of the "vis a tergo" was absorbed at those two sites. The residual pressure was thence directed backward and downward to be met by the wider and longer human sacrum, and the rearranged levator ani muscle which now both filled in bony deficiencies and was adapted as a sphincter for the emerging urethra, vagina and anal canal (see frontispiece).

Inferiorly the human female vagina is supported strongly where it traverses the urogenital diaphragm. This anatomy is similar in the quadruped, and also in both animal and human the vagina above this relative fixation is characterized by free mobility. In the animal, mobility persists into the upper vagina and uterus, for dissection shows upper vaginal and uterine supporting tissues are flimsy and mechanically worthless. The erect human attitude has required change and evolution has produced various thickenings in retroperitoneal tissues most notably that related to the vascular bundle originating from the lateral pelvic wall. The characteristic of the human vagina therefore is fixity above due to the parametrial tissues whose presence sites the upper genital tract over the levator plate in an almost horizontal position, and fixity below at the levator hiatus with marked mobility between. Additionally the human levator ani shows marked differences from the ruminant animal, the principal features being the thick and well developed levator plate and thickened levator crura and the more laterally one moves from these two sites, the more the muscle diminishes, to be replaced by fascia, suggesting strongly that the major work is performed in these two sites. This anatomy is true for the Occidental female, but in other racial groups, notably the Oriental, the muscle is much better developed throughout its entire extent.

After surgical conversion to female genital anatomy, male transsexual patients are not prone to invert the neovagina despite the fact it is not fixed over and to the levator plate. Vaginal examination of such patients at a transsexual clinic in Singapore (Ratnam, 1981) suggests that the strong male levator complex is the probable reason, for the levator hiatus is much narrower in the male, and the strong crural contraction effectively closes off the hiatal defect to prevent any possibility of vault inversion. Additionally some young Asian females have been able to develop the levator crura to such a degree that the retention of fluid or solid objects within the vagina can be demonstrated in certain nightclubs in the East.

Aetiology

Genital prolapse may be considered as the end result of imbalance between intra-abdominal pressure on one hand, and the anatomical structures which support the genital tract on the other. After argument spread over many years, the manner of genital tract support presently advocated finds fairly general acceptance. Relatively fixed at its upper and lower ends, the human vagina enjoys mobility between these points, and the effect of the upper tethering arrangement is to site the vagina and upper genital tract over the anococcygeal raphe of the levator ani muscle complex — the levator plate.

Many local and general factors may have a role to play in the genesis of prolapse but most significant are those which raise intra-abdominal pressure or have a direct weakening effect upon the anatomical supports of he genital tract. Local factors, either congenital or acquired in origin exert their effect upon the genital tract supports whereas general factors, in the main, have to do with an increase in intra-abdominal pressure.

Local Factors

i) Congenital

Congenital defects may affect the pouch of Douglas, the nerve supply to the levator ani group of muscles, or the connective tissue of the pelvic cellular tissue complex.

Daniel Fiske-Jones (1916) writing on the possible role of a deep cul-de-sac in the production of genital and rectal prolapse, observed that the pelvic fascia from its attachment at the pelvic brim, swept down and in toward the bladder, then split to enclose the vagina and attach to the cervix, where it helped form the vaginal vault. He believed this strong fibrous sling was the main bladder support and the strongest uterine support. The posterior part of the fascia was deeper than the anterior, and attached intimately to the rectal wall. A defect in the fascia was responsible for an extension of the cul-de-sac down to the levator muscles and also he believed a deep posterior cul-de-sac was essential to the formation of perineal, rectal and vaginal herniae. Meigs (1947) considered true enterocoele to be a small, narrow, thin-walled sac, probably congenital in origin, which formed directly behind the cervix and lay between the posterior vaginal wall, and the anterior rectal wall and rectovaginal septum. The sac originated behind the cervix between the uterosacral ligaments and was overlooked easily at laparotomy, so Meigs' custom was to lift the uterus high and forward, observing and palpating with his forefinger in the area between the uterosacrals, where often a small dimple — an incipient enterocoele — could be detected. He classed this type of hernia not as a prolapse of the cul-de-sac; but as a separate hernia of congenital type.

Austin and Damstra (1957) proposed a congenital basis for the development of enterocoele, but considered descent of small intestine into a cul-de-sac, either or shallow or deep, could not be classed as hernia, unless a peritoneal defect was present permitting an outpouching of small intestine into the vagina, rectum or perineal body. They related "the prolapse syndrome" to tissue quality and applied it to 67 women who developed an enterocoele, after amassing a group total of 283 pelvic operations, the most common being vaginal hysterectomy.

Congenital defects involving nerve supply of the levator complex have been mentioned often, and the literature contains frequent examples of an association between congenital prolapse and spina bifida. Findley (1917) commenting on the association of virginal uterine prolapse and spina bifida, noted the relationship was interpreted either as faulty innervation of all supporting structures, or of the uterine ligaments in particular. Cases of prolapse in newborn were cited where lack of muscle tone due to defective innervation was present, to add weight to the theory that intra-abdominal pressure was resisted by an uterus supported by muscular structures alone. Torpin (1942) and Cottom and Williams (1965) reported on the aetiological role of spina bifida and noted particularly that involved lower sacral nerve roots meant weakness or paralysis of pelvic floor muscles. Ajabour (1976) writing on genital prolapse in newborn noted previous papers which indicated the close relationship to spina bifida, yet his patient with congenital prolapse did not, and he suggested that congenital elongation of the cervix with secondary prolapse and congenital weakness of the pelvic floor, could be contributory factors.

Congenital defects in pelvic cellular tissues are blamed often as a cause of genital prolapse and although a commonly held view, in fact there is little factual supporting evidence. Stoddard and Meyers (1968) indicated that prolapse was more common in women with generalised connective tissue disorders, and believed a basic defect was the organization of collagen bundles into defective "wickerwork" with disturbed molecular attachments. Recurrent pelvic floor relaxations were common in such patients with inherited connective tissue disorders, and in addition, such patients might give a history of recurrent post-partum haemorrhage, ecchymoses, petechiae, metrorrhagia, cerebral haemorrhage, varicose veins, spontaneous abortion and prematurity. The defect was believed to be change in the amino-acid sequence of collagen, the difference in location of only one amino-acid in the collagen molecule, causing a complete alteration to the "wickerwork". Accordingly they suggested the use of foreign materials e.g. mersilene, teflon, as an adjunct to prolapse repair in patients with suspected connective tissue disorders. El-Kholi and Mina (1975) studied elastic tissue fibres of the vagina in 48 women of different age groups, both with and without prolapse and found they were minimal with marked fragmentation in multiparous menopausal women, and markedy reduced with cystocoele. It was their opinion that changes in vaginal elastic tissue could be the initial lesion in some cases of genital prolapse. Al-Rawi and Al-Rawi (1982) commented on the association of prolapse with joint hypermobility, in a study which showed increased joint laxity in such patients. Their patients were younger than usual, probably due to earlier marriage and motherhood quite usual in their society. Obesity featured in both studies, and backache was recorded twice as often in those with prolapse. Holland (1972) believed the inevitable loss of elasticity in supporting connective tissue was accentuated by improper surgical techniques which failed to support the upper vagina after hysterectomy, and enunciated four basic surgical principles to avoid this error. Approximation of the uterosacral and cardinal ligaments in the midline was vital, with obliteration of the cul-de-sac, then fixing the vaginal vault to these reconstituted ligaments and utilising the paravaginal supporting tissues above the levator muscles, were his key steps. He concluded by approximating levator fascia at the middle third of the vagina. Undoubtedly large pulsion enterocoele occurs most commonly following pelvic surgery of various types and perhaps the reasons given by Holland might be the important ones.

ii) Acquired

Many consider that pregnancy and labour constitute most important aetiological factors, the frequency of prolapse increasing with rising parity, also factors other than parity are decisive particularly large babies and inadequate management of labour. With the onset of pregnancy, the balance between intra-abdominal pressure and genital tract supports is disturbed. Pressure rises and the supports soften, the situation being accentuated by the antigravity position, large baby, multiple pregnancy, obesity etc. Even without the effect of gravity in sheep, the softening of pregnancy probably is a critical factor in prolapse development. Following delivery, the ability of the patient's tissues to involute to prepregnancy dimensions is a vital characteristic in deciding whether or not any deficit remains and it is this quality inherent in her tissues, modified by any degree of congenital deficiency which will decide the completeness of involution. Should any deficit persist, the effects of time and oestrogen deprivation, gravity, obesity, chronic cough, constipation and especially repeated pregnancy eventually may lead to prolapse. Undoubtedly problems at delivery will add to the likelihood of eventual prolapse development, but incomplete involution is the primary defect.

Taylor (1966) commented on a matter of interest and importance in the failure of Caesarean section to prevent recurrent prolapse, for undoubtedly pregnancy weakened the pelvic floor by softening pelvic tissues and stretching them when the presenting part lay in the pelvis in late pregnancy. Damage was caused by pregnancy rather than delivery, and providing a patient's pelvic floor was given the same treatment post-delivery as after vaginal repair surgery possibly there would be less need for repeat repair procedures.

Timonen et al. (1968) noted a high proportion of prolapse in women delivered at home. Probably a prolonged second stage of labour caused stretching of the urogenital hiatus and prolapse development which they believed would have been minimised by operative intervention. There have been many reports of damage to the levator muscle during parturition (Berglas and Rubin, 1953, and Porges et al., 1960). Reports have included damage to puborectalis which was overstretched and torn frequently, particularly fibres which passed around the posterior aspect of the vagina to terminate anterior to the rectum. A more subtle change was separation of the anterior fibres of puborectalis from their insertion at the symphysis and pubic ramus, since such traumatic lacerations were followed by devitalisation, muscle atrophy and fibrous tissue replacement. Should the crural margins separate widely, the anterior vaginal wall would sag between them, and leave the way open for the development of cystocoele, despite compensatory vesicovaginal fibrous thickening. A further change that levator might undergo, possibly unrelated to trauma was manifested by generalised atrophy and thinning, producing a funnel-like descent of the entire pelvic floor and in such instances the levator could lose its ability to contract synchronously and synergistically with the anterior abdominal wall.

Power (1946) described the pelvic floor in parturition and showed how the musculofascial plate which enclosed the pelvis was converted to an open funnel, to allow the foetus to pass. As the lower segment expanded during labour, the endopelvic connective tissue attachment to the cervix, widened and flared in a corresponding manner, thereby assuming the capacity to hold the uterus down in the pelvis against a force tending to pull the walls of the uterus and vagina up, a force equal and opposite to the force trying to expel the foetus. Possibly the physiological function of endopelvic connective tissue during labour was to anchor the lower part of the birth canal, and pregnancy primed it for this task by hypertrophy with an increase in vessel calibre in the vascular pedicles. Porges et al. (1960) considered that the genital hiatus rarely resumed normal nulliparous dimensions in parous females so a further mechanism was required to aid uterine support. Enlargement of the hiatus with widening of the introitus, shifted part of the responsibility for uterine support to the anterior vaginal wall, which became an hypertrophied plate-like structure overlapping the lateral crura of the levator muscle, forming an oblique canal with the posterior

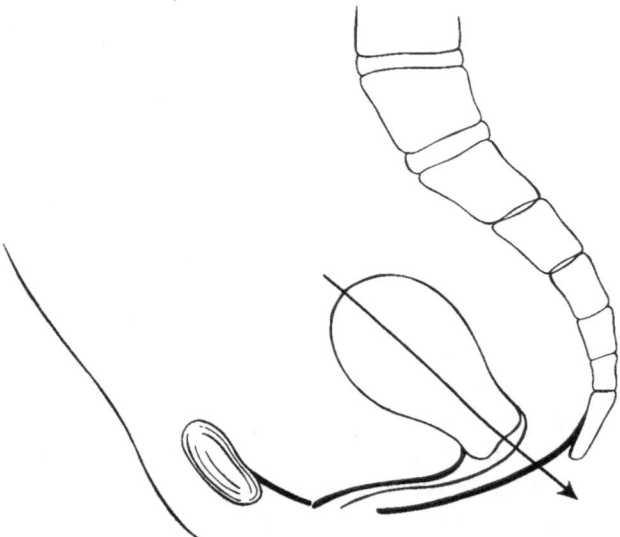

Figure 32. Porges pelvic valve. The heavy lines represent the thickened anterior vaginal wall with pelvic cellular tissue above, and the levator muscle below. (From Porges et al.)

portion of that muscle. Any increase in intra-abdominal pressure caused a valve-like closure of the hiatus, the thickened anterior wall together with the endopelvic connective tissue of the region forming the anterior leaf of what they named "the pelvic valve" (Fig. 32). The posterior leaf of the valve was levator muscle and similar valve mechanisms could be found in other regions such as the inguinal canal. Cox and Webster (1975) reported a high incidence of genital prolapse amongst Pokot women of East Africa, although genital prolapse in other ethnic women was uncommon. Pokot were semi-nomadic, lived on a diet of blood and milk, and all women were circumcised at about 15 years, with marriage following soon after. Babies were delivered in the squatting position in the villages but because of the perineal scars, there was great delay in the second stage of labour. Pushing by the patient helped by strong fundal pressure and an anterior episiotomy which was never sutured, eventually effected delivery. They believed the increased incidence of prolapse in this ethnic group was due to conduct of labour and consequent damage to genital tract supports.

Prophylaxis against damage to genital tract supports during parturition has centred on antenatal physiotherapy with all its benefits in the management of normal labour, the judicious use of forceps delivery, and the advocacy by many of the routine use of episiotomy to lessen levator damage during birth of the foetal head. Undoubtedly all these activities are useful but whether they help in preventing prolapse is difficult to assess.

Surgical damage to the upper vagina resulting either in excessive shortening following reparative vaginal surgery, or greatly increased mobility after abdominal hysterectomy means inadequate support afforded to the upper genital tract by the levator complex (Holland, 1972). Unless the vagina overlies the levator plate, clearly it cannot be supported during a rise in intra-abdominal pressure. Such upper vaginal changes presuppose damage to already tenuous upper vaginal supports. Lack of support will be accentuated if levator function is imperfect. Porges and Porges (1966) commented upon the likelihood of a shortened vagina to invert (Fig. 33) and a normal length vagina with excessive post-surgical mobility has been noted repeatedly during surgical correction of pulsion enterocoele (Zacharin and Hamilton, 1979).

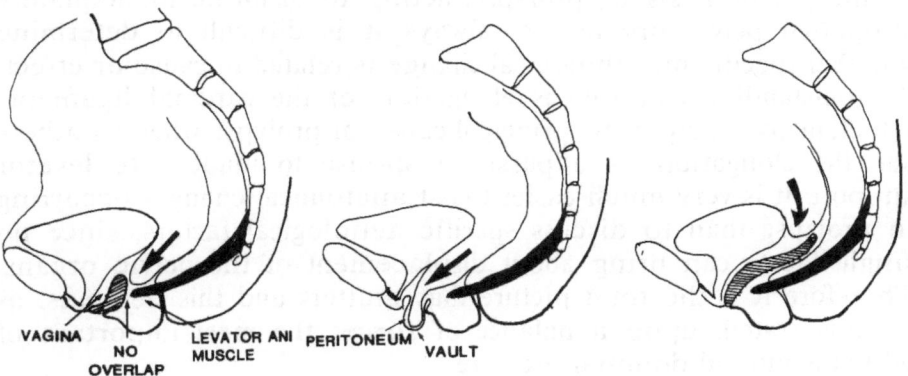

VAGINA LEVATOR ANI PERITONEUM
  NO MUSCLE   VAULT
 OVERLAP

Figure 33. A very short vagina cannot be supported by levator ani and intra-abdominal pressure will cause it to invert. The normal length vagina shown on the right can be supported by the levator. (From Porges and Porges)

General Factors

Intra-abdominal pressure rises are absorbed largely by the anterior abdominal wall, and the bony pelvis due to the lumbosacral curve — a unique human feature. The remainder of the force is then expended against the sacrum, pushing the genital tract and rectum onto the tense levator plate. Since the levator hiatus is well forward in the pelvic outlet, most of the intra-abdominal pressure does not affect it.

Halban and Tandler (1907) stated "the organs of the pelvis and especially the uterus are fixed in their positions by the action of the abdominal pressure. With an elevation in pressure the uterus is pressed firmly against the underlying structures and fixed. By pressing individual organ segments against their underlying structure, the abdominal pressure functions as a factor in fixation, despite its general tendency to dislocate organs".

Common general influences to cause an elevation in intra-abdominal pressure are clearly of great significance and include pregnancy, chronic coughing, chronic constipation and obesity. Elevations of intra-abdominal pressure certainly are an essential factor in the pathogenesis of prolapse, acting to dislocate inadequately supported pelvic organs, yet always it is difficult to determine whether specific morphological change is related to cause or effect. An outstanding example is elongation of the cardinal ligaments which many consider the principal cause of prolapse whereas others see the elongation as a passive response to inadequate levator support. It is very much easier to list anatomical changes occurring in prolapse than to discuss specific aetiological factors, since no single factor can bring about displacement of the pelvic organs. Therefore it is the total picture that matters and this depends, as already stated, upon a balance of forces the most important of which is intra-abdominal pressure.

Ryan (1980) discussing aetiological factors in rectal prolapse considered straining at stool against a closed levator anal sphincter mechanism, produced rectal prolapse rather than faecal incontinence. Such straining could be obsessive on the part of patients with psychological problems and a reduced awareness that their rectum was empty. It could produce rectal intussusception either through a normal pelvic floor, or in the elderly through a weak pelvic floor where supporting tissues of the rectum were defective. Hence the classical abnormalities of deep pouch, unsupported rectum and weak pelvic floor, should be considered as effects rather than causes. It is highly probable that a similar situation could play a role in the onset of genital prolapse.

The combination of rectal prolapse with vault inversion is rare, Emge and Durfee (1966) in their review of the history of prolapse covering 4000 years do not mention the association. Amico and Marino (1968) reported their own case and only one other but Azpuru (1974) reported 5 patients where the problems were combined and a further 12 where rectal prolapse followed a corrected genital prolapse by some years. Neither paper offered any explanation for either the cause or rarity of the association, yet presumably defects in both the pelvic cellular tissues and levator complex together with factors increasing intra-abdominal pressure would have been responsible.

Pelvic organs overlying an enlarged levator hiatus are subject to eventual expulsion by intra-abdominal pressure. Bulging of the anterior vaginal wall will occur if the medial edges of puborectalis separate too widely, and cystocoele results from decompensation in this area. Similarly does a rectocoele form. Loss of muscle mass and reduction of tone in the levator causes still greater pelvic floor obliquity with increased hiatal dimensions, also diminution of uterine size with advancing years allows less of it to derive support from the levator complex. It may be presumed therefore that elongation and stretching of parametrial tissues is secondary. Porges described two distinct types of prolapse. In the first the levator was funnelled with a steep, oblique, vertical course, and the hiatus enlarged secondarily. Here the cervix formed the first part of the prolapse. In the second type, where the cervix came last, the main defect existed in the anterior portion of the hiatus where a primary cystocoele led an even greater part of the pelvic viscera over the genital hiatus. Malpas (1955) believed uterovaginal prolapse represented connective tissue failure whilst general prolapse probably resulted from pelvic floor deficit, particularly levator ani.

Prophylactic therapy may be directed toward the lowering of intra-abdominal pressure by weight control, diagnosis and management of chronic coughing and attention to chronic constipation. Whilst such help will not change an already developed prolapse, the benefit to be gained in terms of minimising later prolapse recurrence following surgery is most certainly very important.

Advancing age, with tissue deterioration accentuated by oestrogen deprivation is a most important general factor since prolapse is seen most commonly in postmenopausal women. However Timonen et al (1968) noted that the onset of a late menarche was common in nulliparous women who developed prolapse after the menopause, and they suggested this early hormonal deficiency might play a more important role than the deficiency due to aging.

Conclusions

When the damaged levator complex loses its ability for synchronous response, undue stress is transmitted to the vascular pedicles which have less capacity to resist, and with the uterus in the vaginal axis the cervix acts as a dilating wedge preventing close apposition of the two elements of the pelvic valve, and this is intussusception. Increased intra-abdominal pressure indirectly fixes the body of the uterus against the posterior aspect of the levator, dislocating the cervix through the open hiatus and constant repetition leads to cervical elongation. The rapidity with which stretching and elongation of the cervix can occur was confirmed clinically by Porges using a Schatz pessary, a dish with multiple perforations. After inserting this pessary for six weeks into a female with prolapse, tongues of cervix protruded slightly through each perforation, indicating clearly that the part of the uterus which overlay the posterior rim of the hiatus would elongate. Cardinal ligaments holding up the uterus failed to explain the phenomenon of cervical elongation. Geary (1972) agreed that the present concept of genital tract support indicated a dual system of ligament and muscle and both were important, for should the musculature be removed, ligamentous support alone could not prevent pelvic visceral prolapse. Conversely, the muscle alone could not prevent prolapse. The two systems were complementary, the cardinal ligaments holding the cervix in a relatively rigid, fixed position back in the pelvis with the fundus in the anterior position, so that intra-abdominal pressure was distributed broadly over endopelvic fascia and pelvic musculature. Nicholls (1969) considered prolapse was caused either by inversion of the upper vagina or eversion of the lower, inversion usually being of post-obstetric origin or due to chronically increased intra-abdominal pressure. Straining inverted the upper vagina but the lower vagina did not evert because eversion resulted from damage to pelvic and urogenital diaphragms with loss of support for the lower vagina, and although occasionally post-obstetric more commonly it was associated with post menopausal atrophy. When both conditions occurred together, the vagina both inverted from above and everted from below.

Thickening of the vascular pedicles appears as a compensatory antigravity effect since it is absent in fourfooted animals. Levator ani is thickened primarily at the anococcygeal raphe and crura, the assumption being that the brunt of the remaining force of intra-abdominal pressure is accepted in these two areas. Berglas and Rubin changed functional anatomical thinking when they examined living females, for past decisions had been taken on cadavers and levator myography showed how the muscle functioned in the intact living female and pointed up its defects in women with prolapse. Furthermore it explained why the anococcygeal raphe — the levator plate — and the crura were the best developed regions. So genital tract support is supplied by the levator plate providing the muscle is undamaged and able to tense in response to intra-abdominal pressure. There is adequate documented evidence about types of levator damage that may be sustained following pregnancy and parturition. The relative inflexibility of undamaged upper genital tract supports — vascular pedicles and connective tissue — sites the uterus and upper vagina over the levator plate.

So the important aetiological factors are those which lead to rises in intra-abdominal pressure or damage to the levator ani/pelvic cellular tissue mechanism. Intra-abdominal pressure may be raised dramatically by pregnancy, obesity, cough or constipation and obsessive straining. The trauma of pregnancy necessarily leaves a mark on the levator muscle of every female, prominent sites being the crura and the bony origin of the muscle from the pubic bones. The primary taint of defective post-pregnancy involution together with such levator damage probably decides "whether" a prolapse will develop; but it is the summation of repeated pregnancy, gravity, time and post menopausal atrophy, chronic cough, obesity and heavy duties grafted onto this background that will decide "when".

Dissections of the Oriental female pelvis indicate that a deep pouch of Douglas alone is unlikely to lead to enterocoele. Kuhn and Hollyock (1982) examined 44 Occidental women to establish a normal range for dimensions of the rectovaginal pouch and rectovaginal septum in nulliparas and ascertain the effect of parturition on these measurements. They found that neither parturition nor prolapse changed the depth of the pouch and furthermore no relation between pouch depth and the presence of enterocoele was detected.

More likely the anatomical defects described above, enhanced by pelvic surgery, allow intra-abdominal pressure, itself accentuated by many accessory factors, to produce the vaginal inversion. It is evident there are two types of genital prolapse, each at the opposite end of the spectrum of anatomic defects, with the more common variety regarded as vaginal intussusception, the cervix being the intussuscipiens, and thereby akin to rectal prolapse which general consensus today regards as intussusception. Ripstein (1963) believed rectal prolapse resulted from the rectum being displaced forwards from the sacral hollow either by the possession of a congenital defect — the mesorectum — or in the elderly by stretching and atrophy of normal rectal supports. So the rectum overlay the levator hiatus. The mechanism of prolapse, once rectal displacement had occurred was the same in both groups. Increased intra-abdominal pressure acting in the long axis of the bowel ultimately produced a sliding hernia through the anterior defect in the pelvic floor; but since the anus was relatively fixed in position, the bowel intussuscepted. As secondary effects a large peritoneal sac formed and the anal sphincter began to stretch.

In both problems the accompanying enterocoele sac can be regarded as secondary, and termed traction. There is little true uterine descent in this type of genital prolapse, merely gross cervical hypertrophy and elongation. Traction enterocoele with genital prolapse usually is not large, and prolapse correction is followed only rarely by pulsion enterocoele. One may presume that both pelvic cellular tissues and levator complex are functioning well. At the other end of the spectrum is the less common prolapse, in which defective cellular tissues and levator ani have allowed widening of the levator hiatus, relaxation of fascial support to the upper vagina, and its anterior displacement over the hiatus. A large peritoneal cul-de-sac results from increased intra-abdominal pressure, which pushes the cervix, upper vagina and attached pouch of Douglas through the widened pelvic aperture inverting the genital tract. Here there is no cervical elongation or hypertrophy, and in this group, no matter what precautions are taken at primary reparative surgery, recurrent pulsion enterocoele is now more likely, for the stage has been set by the underlying anatomic defects.

The Clinical Features of Enterocoele

Classification

There has been much confusion with enterocoele nomenclature in the past ever since first descriptions by de Garengeot (1743) and Astley Cooper (1804). Gaillard Thomas (1885) presented a comprehensive classification of hernias appearing in the vagina or vulva and included "vaginal enterocoele or hernia, meaning the descent of a small portion of small intestine into the vagina". Pudendal or perineal enterocoele similarly was applied to small bowel descent into the labium majus or perineum and these two groups were further subdivided depending upon the contents of the sac. Vaginal hernia, declared by Sweetser (1919) to be a great rarity, found an exit either anterior or posterior to the broad ligament, the anterior hernia descending between the broad ligament and bladder to push the anterior vaginal wall forward, whilst the posterior perforated part of the levator muscle pushing forward the posterior vaginal wall. Miles (1926) suggested pelvic hernia as an inclusive term for all herniae passing through the pelvic floor, and subvarieties were named by their point of egress to be consistent with best usage in hernia nomenclature. Miles subdivisions were pudendal, perineal and vaginal; the latter being split further into anterior or posterior, depending upon the relationship of the sac to the uterus with the anterior vaginal hernia following the cleavage plane between bladder and anterior vaginal wall. The term "levator hernia" (Chase, 1922) could not be applied to all pelvic herniae, since midline herniae passed anterior or posterior to the uterus and did not traverse the levator muscle or fascia. Wilensky and Kaufman (1940) proposed an all-encompassing classification of pelvic herniae, in an endeavour to finalise the situation, and employed the following headings:

1. Extraperitoneal vaginal herniae.
    a) Urethrocoele
    b) Cystocoele
    c) Rectocoele
2. Peritoneal vaginal herniae.
    a) Anterior
    b) Posterior
    c) Lateral anterior
    d) Lateral posterior
    e) Postoperative
3. Perineal hernia
4. Hydrocoele
5. Pudendal hernia
6. Pelvic quasi-herniae
    a) Marked uterine prolapse
    b) Marked rectal prolapse

This classification was much too fussy and quite impractical since it attempted to cover every eventuality, so lost the very necessary ingredient of workable simplicity. Read (1951) divided vaginal enterocoele into two distinct varieties with practical significance. Pulsion enterocoele resulted from intra-abdominal pressure acting upon a congenitally elongated sac, or one elongated purely as a result of thrust from above in association with weak supports below. Traction enterocoele was a frequent accompaniment of uterine or rectal prolapse, being merely a secondary effect produced by the genital or rectal prolapse, whereas pulsion enterocoele was primary and followed the combination of intra-abdominal pressure and weakness in genital tract supports. Nicholls (1972) made the important point that enterocoele with inversion of the vaginal vault, must be distinguished from enterocoele without vault inversion since surgical correction of each was different. Ranney (1980) grouped all these pelvic defects as cul-de-sac relaxations or defects, subdividing them into pelvic hernia, enterocoele and total vaginal prolapse. Pelvic hernia was a narrow-necked deep pouch of peritoneum discovered at laparotomy, mostly medial to the uterosacral ligaments, presumably the "incipient enterocoele" of Meigs. Enterocoele and vaginal prolapse contained many overlapping examples. "Large enterocoeles" bulged to or through the introitus when the labia were separated and the patient strained, "medium sized" usually were symptomless and could be detected during recto-vaginal examination when the patient strained, and a soft balloon was palpable between the index and middle fingers whereas "small or incipient enterocoeles" he emphasised, were often suspected, but not identified until laparotomy. Symmonds and Pratt (1959) recognized three enterocoele types. The simplest developed behind a well-supported anterior vaginal wall usually after vaginal hyster-ectomy, and represented a neglected enterocoele sac — a real or potential sac not recognized during surgery — and a rectocoele may or may not be associated. The second and most common included moderate vault prolapse together with enterocoele, some cystocoele and rectocoele, and the third was total vaginal eversion.

As a practical classification the following is suggested:

Genital Prolapse

Prolapse is of two main types with a spectrum of change between the extremes. The common genital prolapse includes in varying degree of severity and differing combinations, cystocoele, cervical hypertrophy and elongation, traction enterocoele and rectocoele. Usually there is no real uterine descent, vault prolapse being apparent only, due to cervical elongation, and in large measure, genital tract supports are intact so pulsion enterocoele will be an unlikely late complication following repair procedures (Fig. 34).

The less common genital prolapse is a pulsion enterocoele pre-dominantly. There is no cervical elongation, and the vaginal vault descends as a piston, whereas the common prolapse characteristi-cally unwinds about the subpubic arch (Fig. 35). Following repar-ative surgery, since the genital tract supports — levator ani and pelvic cellular tissues — are defective, pulsion enterocoele is much more likely as a late complication. Malpas (1955) drew a distinction between general prolapse with considerable peritoneal herniation but no cervical elongation, and uterovaginal prolapse with elon-gation of the supravaginal cervix, and little enterocoele.

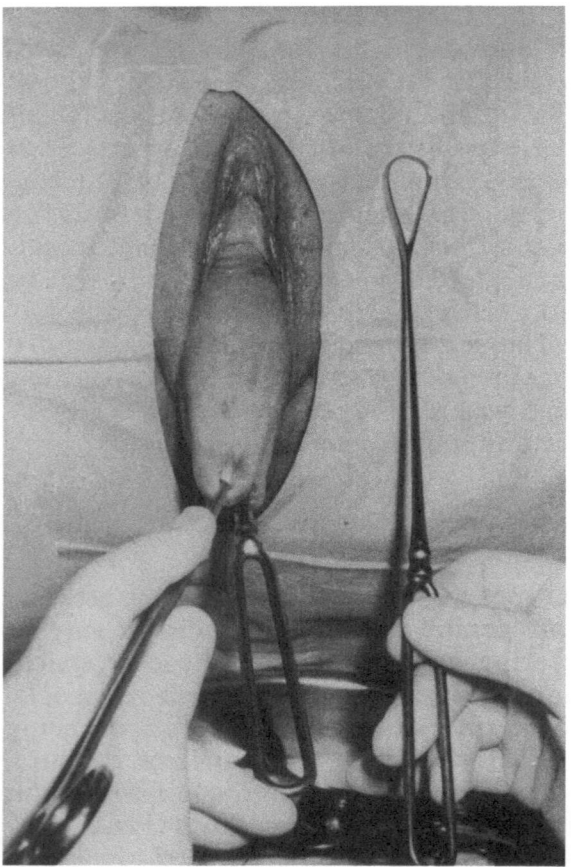

Figure 34. The more common variety of genital prolapse showing the pronounced cervical elongation and hypertrophy

Pulsion Enterocoele

The problem may be small, moderate or large. Smaller defects (the incipient enterocoele) appear through the posterior vaginal wall high up, and characteristically the sac has a relatively narrow neck. There is no associated vault inversion and most probably the cause is a defect in the rectovaginal septum. Large pulsion enterocoele (Syn. inverted vagina) is associated always with vault inversion, the

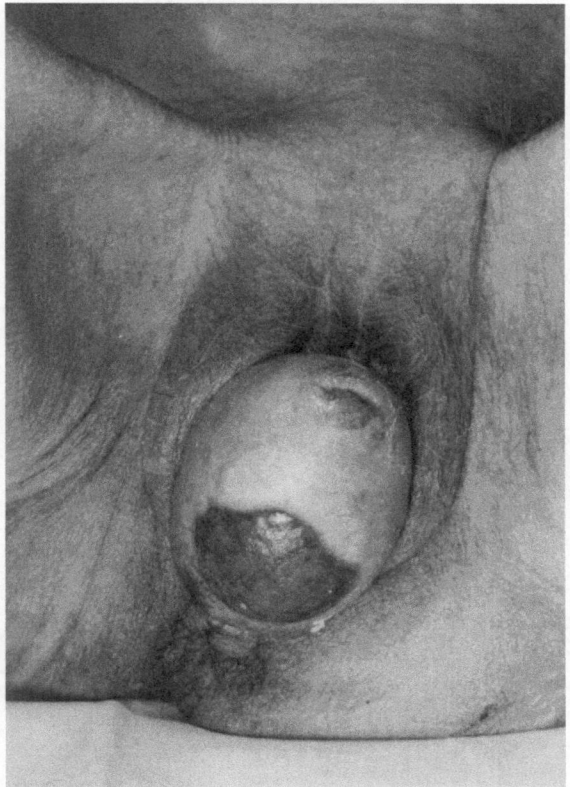

Figure 35. The less common variety of genital prolapse with true genital tract descent and associated large pulsion enterocoele. There is also a large area of decubitus ulceration present posteriorly

underlying cause being defective genital tract supports. Following hysterectomy, either abdominal or vaginal, further damage to already damaged pelvic cellular tissue supports is unavoidable and the stage is set for enterocoele recurrence.

Pudendal or Perineal Hernia

Named for its point of exit, such a hernia appears in the greater labium or perineum, protruding between the muscles or fascia which form the pelvic floor. Pudendal hernia was termed levator hernia by Chase (1922) who proposed a classification and nomen-

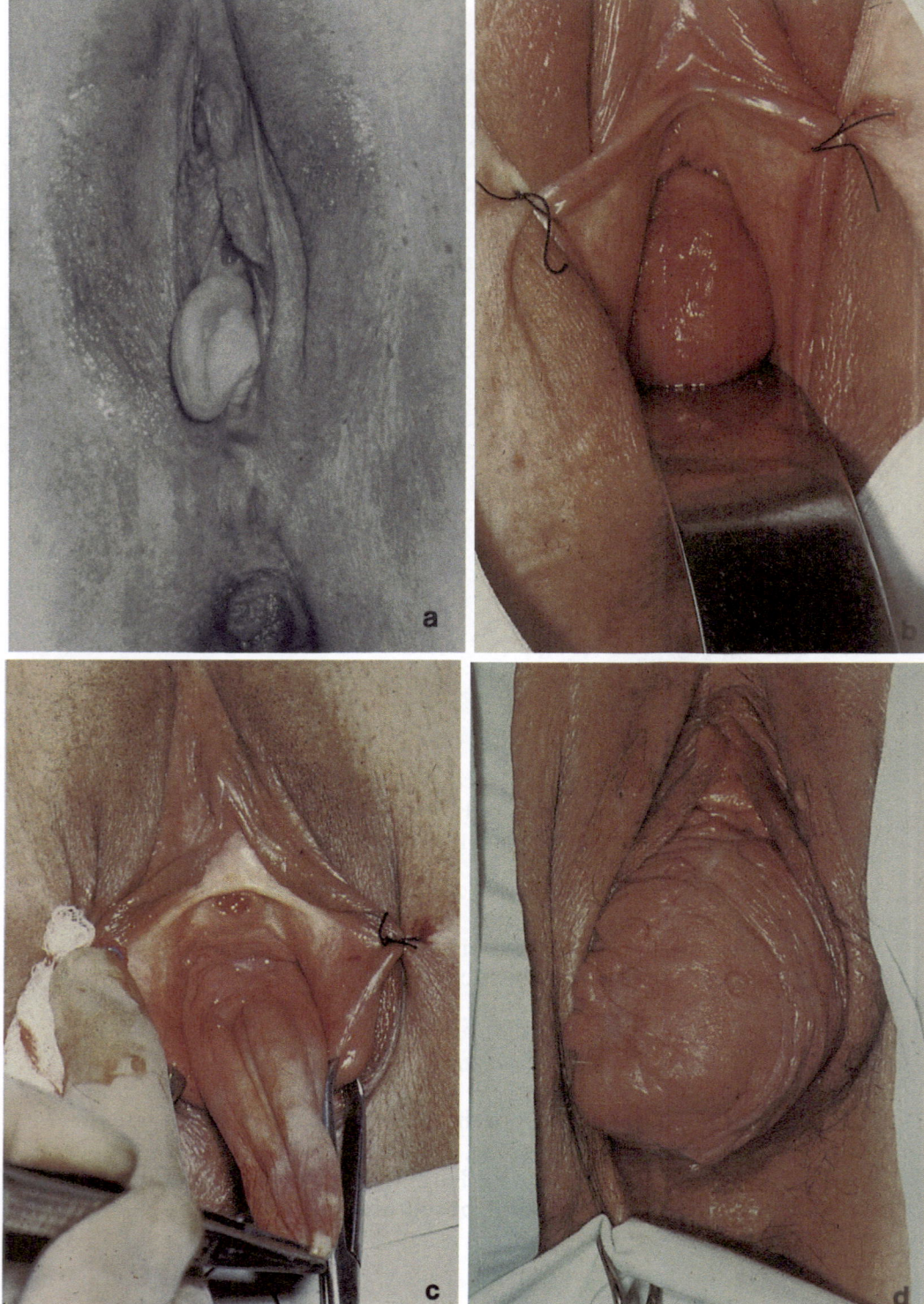

clature based on the anatomical fact that all varieties passed through a levator muscle defect, and he divided them into congenital and acquired, and upon their relation to the broad ligament. Congenital defects in the form of anomalous openings between the pelvic floor muscles or a deep cul-de-sac were believed to be common reasons for their occurrence (Koontz, 1951).

Clinical Picture

Although uncommon, large pulsion enterocoele certainly is not a rarity. The present series is concerned with 122 cases. It occurs as a serious late complication following a variety of pelvic surgical procedures, and is unusual apart from this clinical setting. The greatest frequency is seen following vaginal hysterectomy, and indeed these are the largest hernias which occur. Also it may follow abdominal hysterectomy or the Manchester operation.

The neck of the sac usually is large, and once herniation has been initiated the tendency is to enlarge rapidly. At a variable interval following pelvic surgery, the patient becomes aware of a painless, reducible mass which appears in the vagina, or at the introitus when she stands or strains (Fig. 36a, b, c, d). Often a pressure feeling in the vagina is noted early in the development of the hernia, without other symptoms. Occasionally there may be minor bowel or bladder upsets, rectified by digital pressure on the lump, and when larger by its manual reposition. Weed and Tyrone (1949) and Kinzel (1960) considered the chief symptoms apart from protrusion were referable to the rectum, and included fullness, inability to defaecate, dissatisfaction and even impaction, but such symptoms have been most uncommon in this present series of patients. With enlargement, the usual change at the fundus of the protrusion is abrasion and inflammation caused by trauma from clothing, or when in the sitting position — decubitus ulceration. Early on, a thin rather purulent discharge occurs, but later ulceration appears and frank bleeding results, so that in practice a vaginal protrusion, discharge and bleeding, are the common presenting symptoms (Fig. 37).

Figure 36 a—d. Moderate and large pulsion enterocoeles which followed vaginal hysterectomy

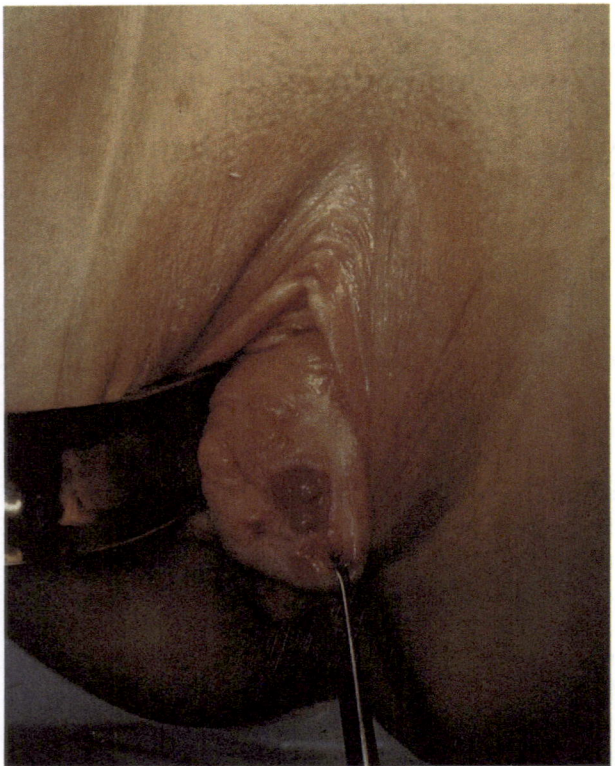

Figure 37. Ulceration occurring at the fundus of a pulsion enterocoele

Diagnosis

With a large defect usually there is no difficulty deciding that pulsion enterocoele is the correct diagnosis, but differentiation between a smaller enterocoele and rectocoele can be difficult, and often not resolved completely until displayed at surgery, so the cul-de-sac always must be explored, without fail. The typical past history, associated with a vaginal protrusion that cascades down the vagina from the vault, is quite characteristic. With the patient positioned in the left lateral position, a Sims speculum inserted into the vagina, and a good light, the patient is asked to strain down. The vault and upper posterior vaginal wall begin to invert and descend the vagina. Slowly withdrawing the speculum whilst supporting the anterior vaginal wall with sponge forceps, will demonstrate the defect with clarity. Additionally, supporting the vaginal vault with the forceps during straining, completely eliminates the defect and is an important and characteristic diagnostic feature. Rarely peristalsis in the contained loops may be observed although Bueermann (1932) considered peristaltic waves which coursed over the surface of the sac following digital irritation, pathognomonic of the presence of small intestine within the sac. The vaginal epithelium should be inspected for health, cleanliness, and incipient ulceration. Frank ulceration will be situated at the tip of the fundus or toward the posterior aspect of the bulge, and only rarely would one have doubts about the nature of the ulceration for the ulcer is shallow with an indolent appearance, a yellowish base, the floor is not indurated nor is the edge rolled or unduly hard. Doubts can be resolved quickly by cytology or observance of healing following vaginal packing for 48 hours, so that biopsy is rarely necessary.

Differential Diagnosis

Major differentiation is from rectocoele, and usually this is a straightforward decision. As the speculum is withdrawn gradually, demonstrating the enterocoele, frequently in the lower vagina a transverse sulcus may be seen dividing the enterocoele above from the rectocoele below. Similarly with the sac supported by sponge holders, a request to the patient to strain will demonstrate the rectocoele bulge and with the patient in the dorsal position and a finger in the rectum, one cannot introduce the rectal finger into the enterocoele bulge. Bueermann offered "a constant and typical sign of vaginal hernia". Digital rectal examination demonstrated that the posterior vaginal wall mass was due only partly to anterior bulging of the rectal wall, but when the patient gave a quick, short cough, a protrusion independent of the rectocoele could be seen. The differentiation of rectocoele from enterocoele really is a little academic, for no matter what choice of surgical correction is selected, both must be investigated during that surgery.

When the uterus is present, anterior enterocoele descending between bladder and cervix can be witnessed when the patient strains, aided by judicious use of the sponge holders, supporting

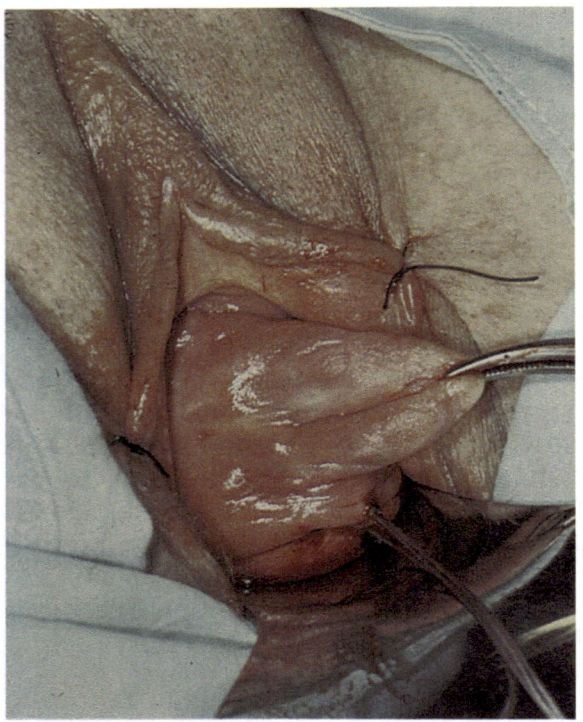

Figure 38 a. Anterior enterocoele. The enterocoele is displayed lying between bladder and cervix

first the cystocoele and later the vault. To be diagnosed, first its presence must be suspected. It is unusual, the only example in this series of patients followed a Manchester operation, and clearly it must have been present prior to surgery. At operation the sac lying between the bladder and cervix was demonstrated clearly (Fig. 38 a, b).

Pudendal and perineal hernia whilst never confused with vaginal enterocoele, nevertheless are similar problems and occasionally have been referred for opinion and management. Essential diagnostic features of pudendal hernia were enumerated by Chase (1922): the hernia appeared in the posterior part of the greater labium, with the medial half of the bulge covered by mucous membrane, the lateral half with integument and the usual signs of hernia were elicited upon examination. Koontz (1951) reported a patient with multiple herniae including a large perineal (buttock) hernia

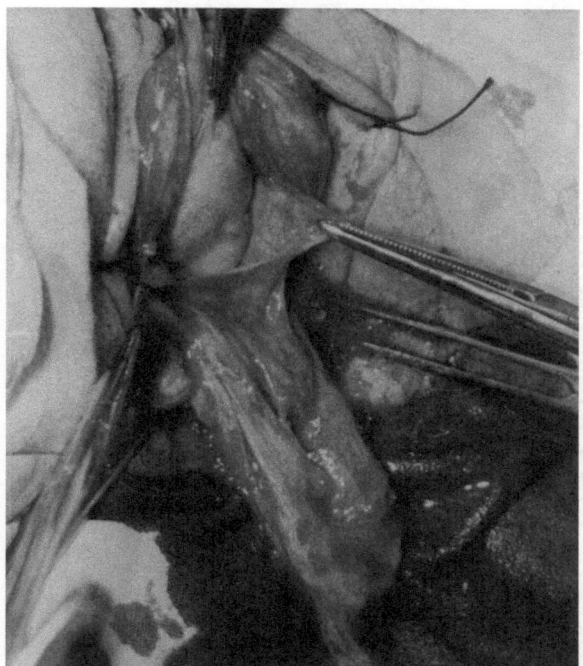

Figure 38 b. Anterior enterocoele. The enterocoele sac opened. The bladder lies above and the reflected anterior vaginal wall skin below

(Fig. 39), and noted the principal types of perineal hernia were anterior and posterior, the anterior traversing the urogenital diaphragm to emerge lateral to the vagina, with the bladder found often in the sac wall being at great risk from any proposed reparative surgery. The posterior perineal hernia emerged in the buttock. In 1951 he found less than 100 reported cases (Fig. 40). Herman (1961) reported a left pudendal hernia and two important observations of great relevance. The first that wrong diagnosis could lead to disastrous surgical results if cyst or abscess was thought to be the problem, and second, many patients because of wrong diagnosis and the assumption that another form of prolapse was present, had been subjected to multiple, useless surgical procedures. His patient, because of her rare problem, had suffered uterine suspension, hysterectomy with removal of both ovaries, vaginal suspension, partial vaginectomy, enterocoele repair, and finally total vaginectomy. He regarded the cause in this case to be probable partial avulsion of the

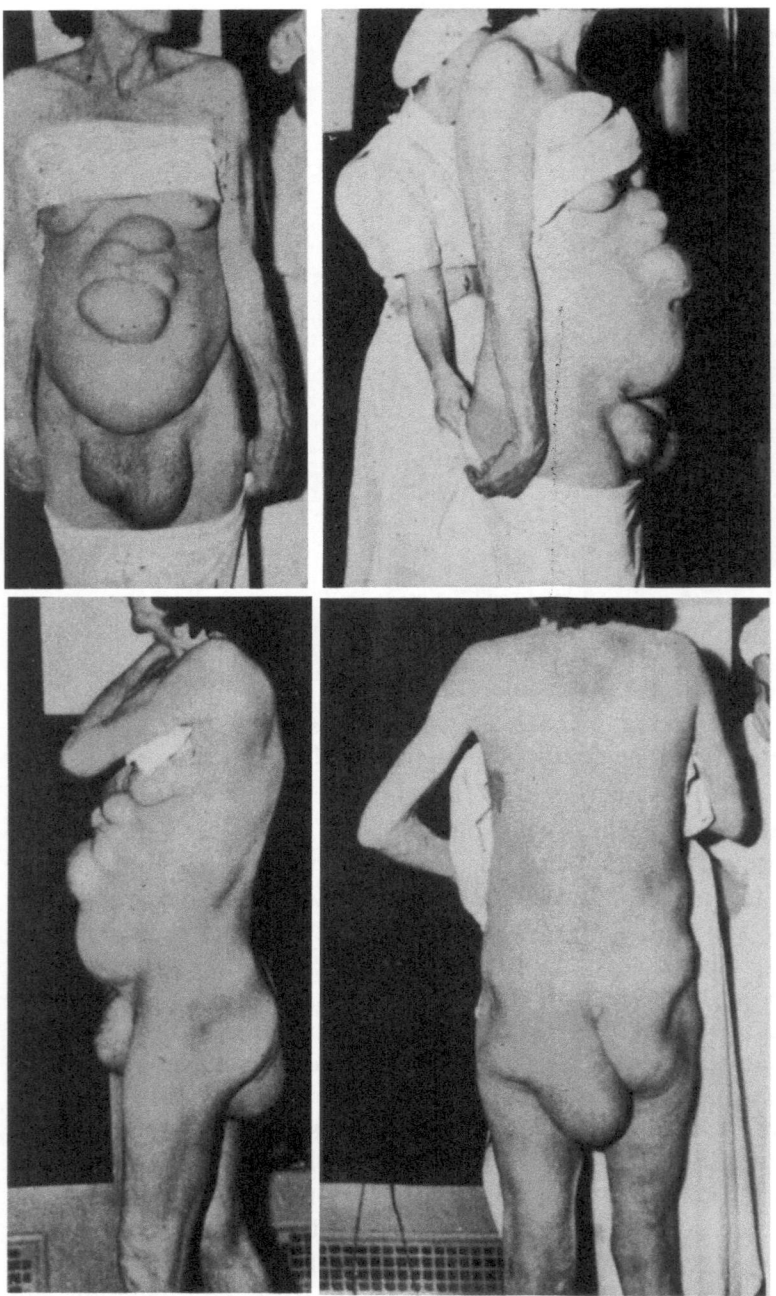

Figure 39. Koontz's patient with multiple herniae, including a large perineal hernia. (From Koontz)

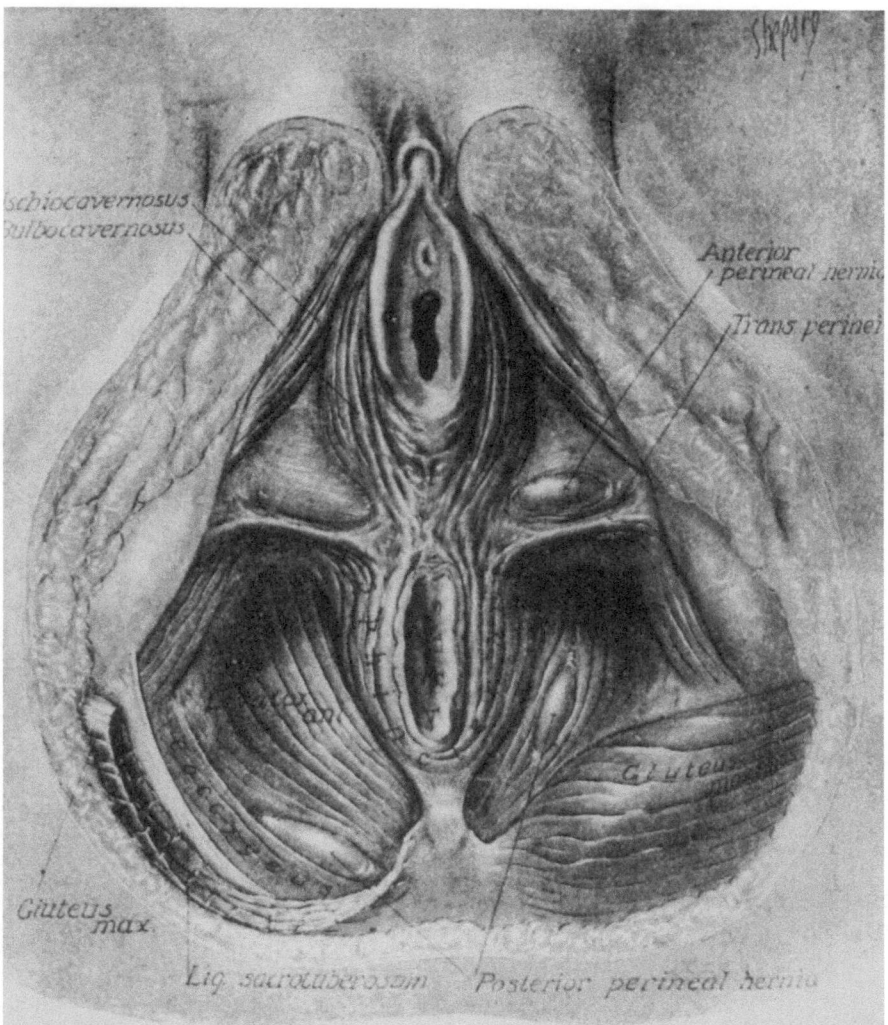

Figure 40. Diagram showing the anatomy of perineal herniae in the female. (From Koontz)

tendinous levator origin from the pelvis during previous surgery. The abdominal approach was advocated as more effective despite the hernia being more obvious from the perineum, although both routes have been mentioned in the literature, and occasionally a combined approach has been employed. At surgery with the right

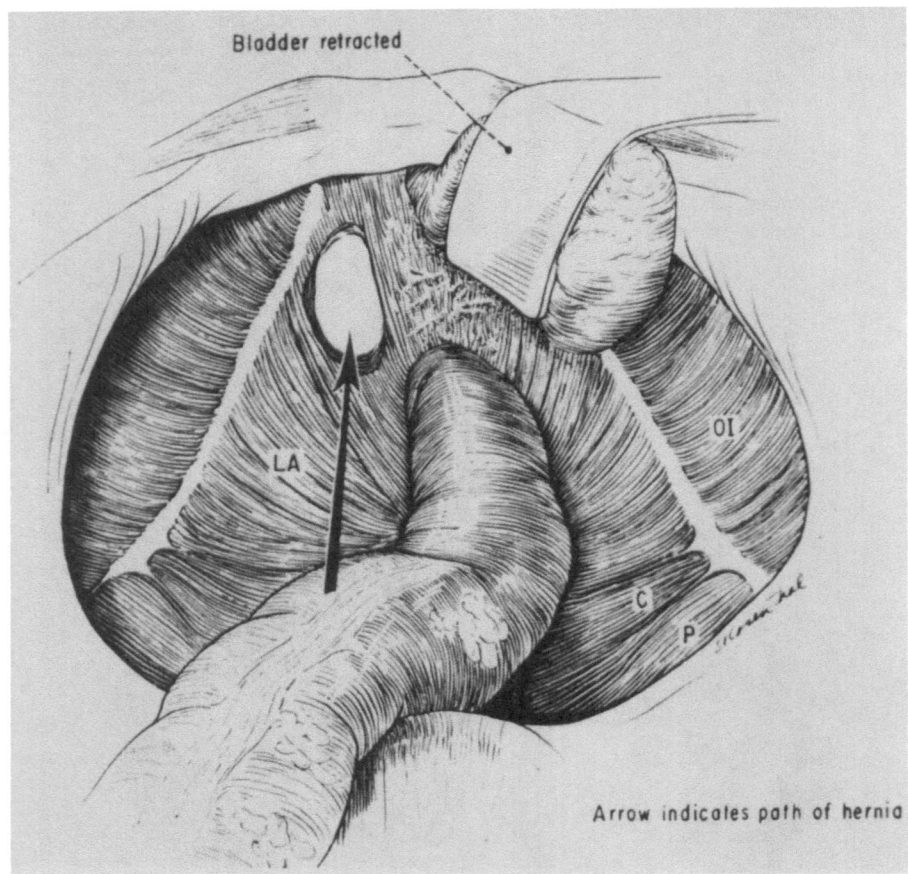

Figure 41. A diagram of the anterior levator defect found at operation. (From Herman)

diagnosis, he found the defect (Fig. 41) and could correct it. He emphasised that irreducibility was the important distinguishing feature of Bartholin or other cyst in the area and inguinal labial hernia when reduced passed over the pelvic brim and into the inguinal canal. Anderson (1968) reported a patient with a misdiagnosed pudendal hernia who encountered a similar surgical fate to Herman's patient. Prior to final diagnosis, she suffered hysterectomy with multiple vaginal repairs, immediate recurrence following the last repair shortly after discharge from hospital and then

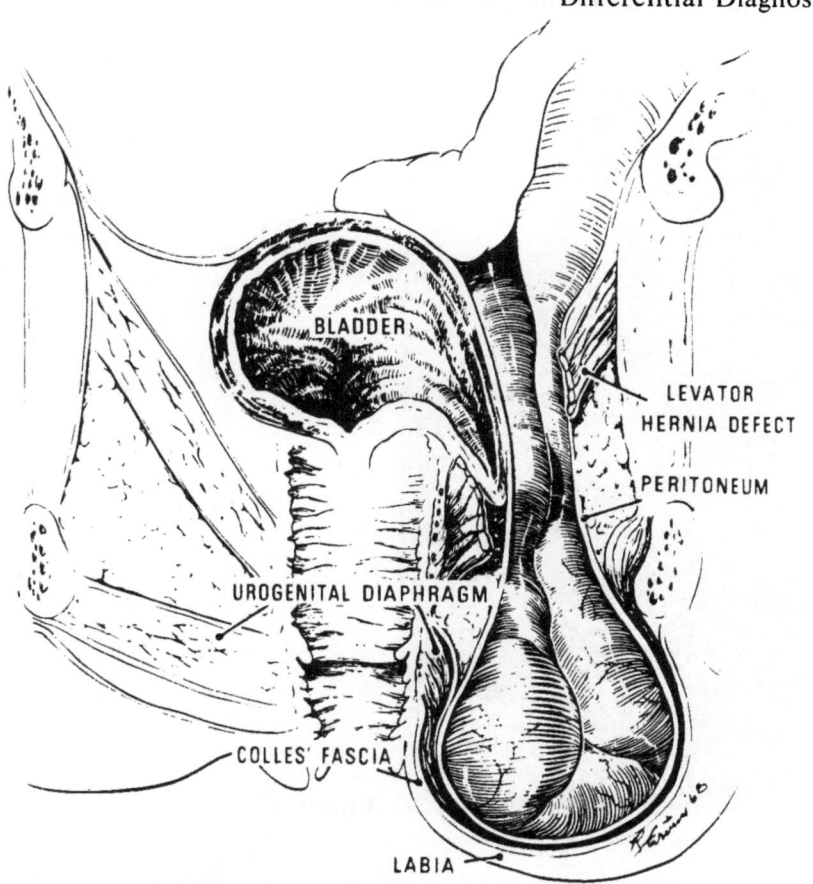

Figure 42. The visceral, muscular and fascial relationships of pudendal hernia. (From Anderson)

another vaginal wall repair one year later which failed also!! Anderson advocated a perineal approach delineating the sac, inverting it and closing the defect with heavy gauge monofilament propylene mesh prior to using levator fascia etc. beneath it. Bladder formed the medial wall of the sac (Fig. 42).

Lash and Levin (1962) suggested X-ray examination with lateral and antero-posterior views of small and large bowel may reveal the true hernial defect present. Fancuilli et al. (1975) reported upon the use of a barium meal to aid in correct diagnosis of vaginal entero-coele and Berg (1979) reported opaque herniography to finalise the diagnosis and again the case which he reported had suffered many surgical onslaughts prior to accurate diagnosis.

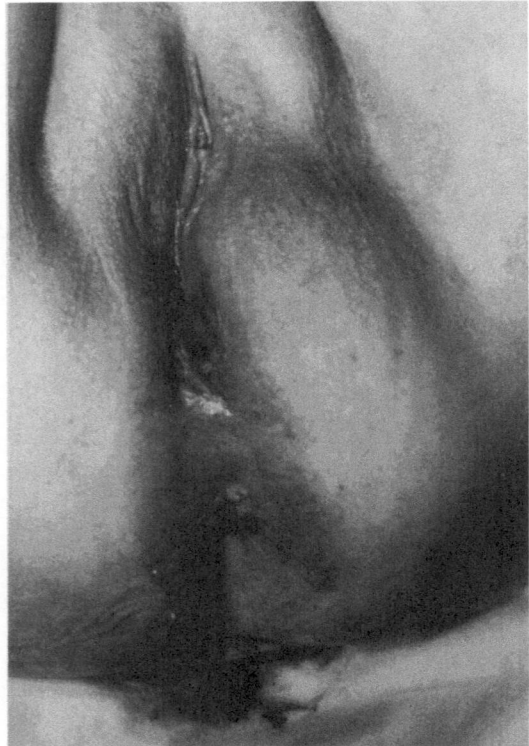

Figure 43 a

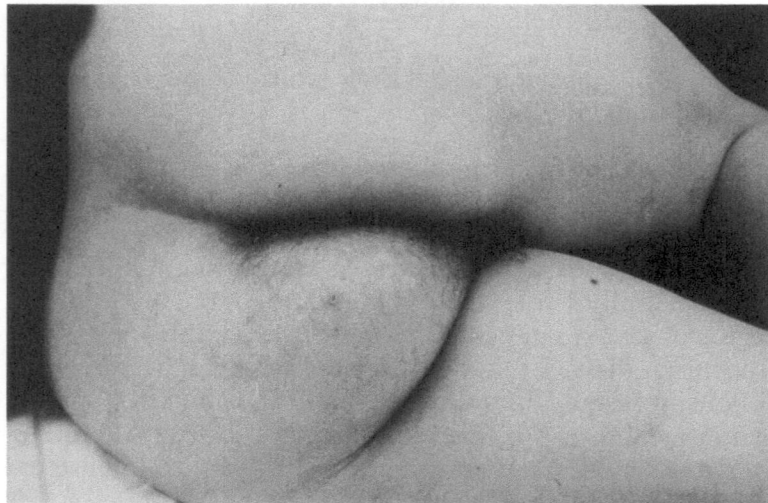

Figure 43 b

Figure 43 a, b. A large left perineal hernia seen in two views

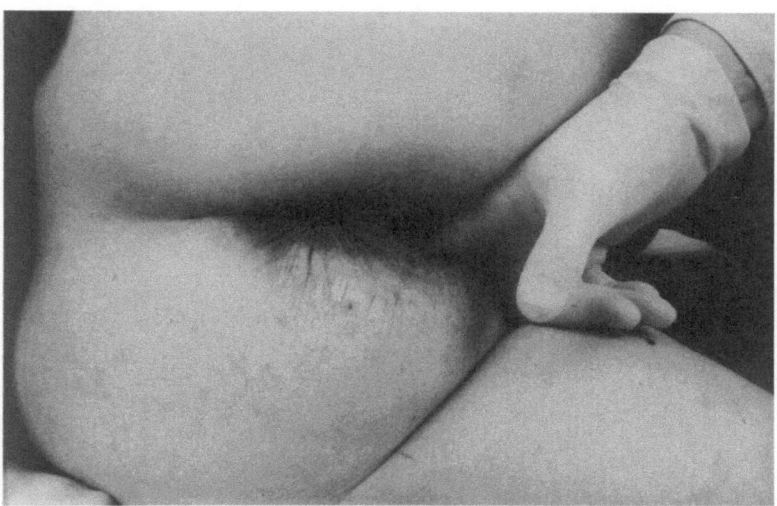

Figure 44. Following reduction of the perineal hernia its descent could be prevented by a finger inserted into the vagina and pressing on the lateral vaginal wall

All perineal herniae presenting in the buttock are not what they seem, even though all the characteristic clinical features of hernia are present. A parous female of 45 years presented with a typical perineal hernia, bulging into the left buttock (Fig. 43 a, b), which had been present for several years and previous laparotomy with attempted sac closure had failed. A large, reducible left buttock mass with a pronounced impulse on coughing presented and vaginal examination showed clearly its pathway down the left lateral vaginal wall. The hernia could be controlled easily with digital pressure (Fig. 44). The features of hernia were so apparent further investigation was thought unnecessary, but ultrasound examination or opaque herniography would have avoided misdiagnosis. The hernia was so large it was feared bladder could form part of its medial wall, for clearly the mass descended lateral to levator ani through the ischiorectal fossa, so a combined synchronous abdominoperineal approach was chosen. The mass was not a hernia, but a large white, soft yet firm and slippery tumour mass sliding down the lateral pelvic wall to appear in the buttock (Fig. 45). Removed in its entirety with many technical problems, the resulting cavity was drained both through the abdomen and vagina. Section showed the tumour to be an aggressive angiomyxoma originating in retroperi-

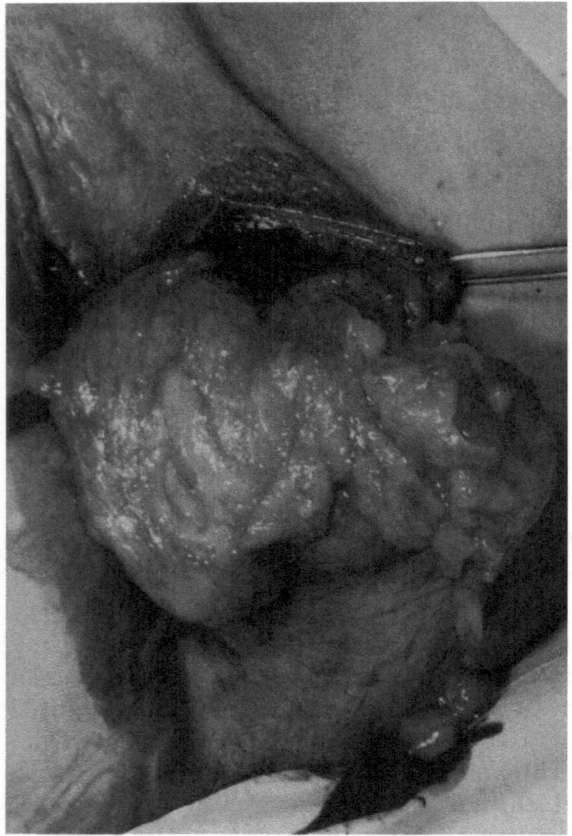

Figure 45. The tumour mass was exposed in the left buttock

toneal tissues. Steeper and Rosai (1983) reported nine cases, and in all the wrong clinical diagnosis had been made.

Complications of Large Pulsion Enterocoele

These are the reasons for advising operative correction of the defect, and depending on the clinical situation the need for surgery may be deferred for a time, or deemed necessary in the near future. The commonest problem is rapid progression in size, with resultant change in the epithelium at the fundus of the hernial sac. Exposure leads to abrasion then infection, ulceration and the likelihood of

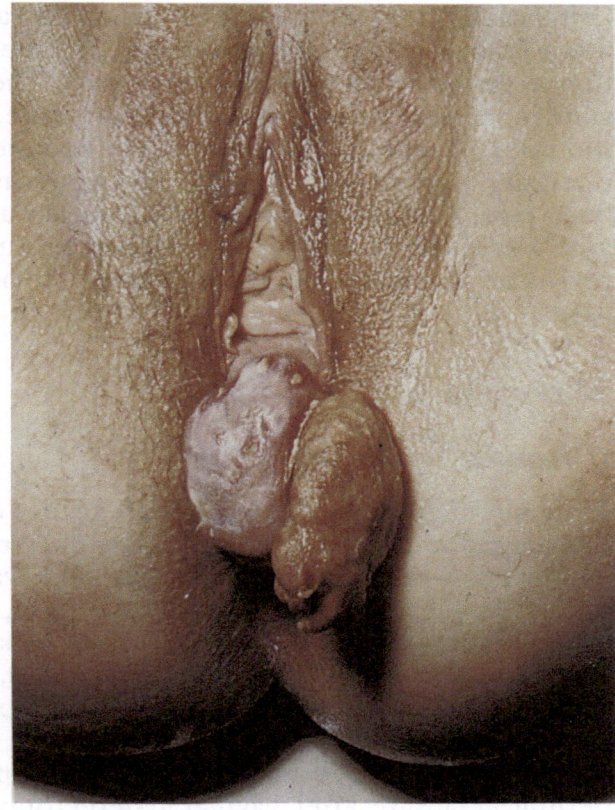

Figure 46. Spontaneous rupture of a large pulsion enterocoele, with the rupture site plugged by omentum

spontaneous rupture either unexpectedly or during straining. Partial rupture may be plugged by a piece of omentum (Fig. 46). Incarceration is rare due to the wide neck of the sac, although Barker (1876) reported a patient who complained of recurrent episodes of intestinal colic relieved by manual reduction of the hernia, and Bueermann (1932) reported such a case with a fatal outcome. The literature suggests incarceration is more likely during labour when the foetal head could impinge on the neck of the sac and prevent reduction of the hernia, which in turn prevents further descent of the presentation. Spontaneous rupture of an enterocoele during straining, with evisceration has been reported by several authors and rarely external violence causing subparietal bowel rupture

(Birchenall, 1869). Powell (1974) found 28 cases of vaginal evisceration following vaginal hysterectomy reported in the literature and they occurred 5—18 months after surgery. The common factor was a sudden increase in intra-abdominal pressure. He commented upon the rarity of rupture compared to the common occurrence of postoperative enterocoele. In addition vault rupture after coitus has been recorded several times and he added a further patient. Chan and Neale (1982) added one case of spontaneous rupture but a review of the literature revealed only 10 other well documented cases.

Management

i) Traction Enterocoele

Traction enterocoele accompanies all grades of genital prolapse and is managed in conjunction with surgical correction of the prolapse. No matter whether Manchester repair or vaginal hysterectomy is employed, the sac always must be explored, and redundancy dealt with appropriately. During Manchester repair, the elongated and enlarged sac should be carefully delineated, opened, and the contents examined, then twisted off as high as possible, transfixed and amputated. The neck is sutured to the back of the cervical stump, hopefully to divert future intra-abdominal pressure thrust. During peritoneal closure after vaginal hysterectomy, many techniques are employed, but the principles are to minimise peritoneal redundancy, and to close the uterosacral space. As indicated previously, if anatomical defects in levator ani and pelvic cellular tissues are such as to be conducive to later pulsion enterocoele development, all precautions taken during vaginal hysterectomy to minimise the likelihood, probably may prove ineffectual.

ii) Pulsion Enterocoele

Management is dictated by the size of the defect, which for practical convenience can be considered as small, moderate or large.

Small pulsion enterocoele, the least common variety, presents as a vaginal swelling some time after previous pelvic surgery. It may be symptomless and found an routine examination, or reach to the introitus yet rarely pass through it to protrude. Examination shows the usual physical signs of pulsion enterocoele, but without associated vault inversion. Probably a small defect in the upper posterior vaginal wall has been responsible for its appearance. The sac neck is narrow and digital palpation shows only a small deficiency. Since small intravaginal pulsion enterocoeles commonly are symptomless, providing the overlying vaginal epithelium is normal in appearance, conservative management is the correct advice. Regular review is required, also the patient is warned of its presence but reassured that no dramatic change is likely. With progression in size or the production of symptoms, surgical correction is required.

The same remarks are true for moderate sized pulsion enterocoele with the following additions. Usually there is some degree of vault inversion, often the lump has begun to protrude through the introitus and commonly early traumatic changes on the covering vaginal epithelium are present. The place for conservative management is less, and advice favouring surgical correction more appropriate. In this present series, large pulsion enterocoele was seen most frequently after vaginal hysterectomy, then abdominal hysterectomy and Manchester repair. Hawksworth and Roux (1958) reported an incidence of 8.5% pulsion enterocoeles occurring in a series of 246 vaginal hysterectomies. Symmonds and Pratt (1960) found 37 of 69 pulsion enterocoeles occurred following vaginal hysterectomy. Embrey (1961) reported a 6% incidence of pulsion enterocoele following vaginal hysterectomy which was much more frequent than after the Manchester operation. However more recent papers have indicated that with improvement in the technique of vaginal hysterectomy, the incidence of late development of enterocoele has been declining (Lee and Symmonds, 1972).

Recurrence may occur quite quickly following surgery (Feroze, 1978), the patient usually complaining of a large bulge presenting at the introitus. Other physiological disturbances are not common. Examination shows typical features with marked vaginal inversion and extensive vault defect indicating the width of the neck of the sac, and often incipient ulceration of the fundus. Questioning indicates that sexual intercourse either has not been resumed since the recent surgery because of the protrusion, or ceased with its appearance. Such a large enterocoele is an urgent surgical problem for it will continue to enlarge rapidly, and because of the ever-present spectre of ulceration and rupture, there can be no place for conservative management.

a) Conservative Management

This method is applicable only when the enterocoele is small and without evident skin changes. Persisting with inaction in the face of rapid enlargement with skin changes is to court disaster. Nicholls (1972) referred to the temporary use of a pessary as non-surgical management in certain types of vault inversion when surgery was inconvenient or contraindicated and Puddington and Guiou (1976) also advocated intravaginal supports of ball and stem or cup and stem types, depending on the presence or absence of the uterus. These authors would be in the minority, and most gynaecologists would regard such management as potentially hazardous. Surgery is the only safe method of management in the face of symptoms or signs of progression and should the patient's general condition be so grave as to completely preclude surgery then she is better left without the pessary — the situation will deteriorate certainly but less quickly than with a pessary.

b) Prophylaxis

Many writers have mentioned general factors which make the likelihood of post-operative pulsion enterocoele greater. It is known that certain races e.g. non-Westernised Chinese, are virtually protected from mechanical problems affecting the pelvic floor because of their superior anatomy and tissue quality (Zacharin, 1977), yet when such Chinese became Westernised — third and fourth generation — the incidence of these problems begins to increase; but not to the level of the Occidental female. It seems that Western influences of obesity, less demanding work, sitting in chairs rather than squatting, and a fairly general level of unfitness are major factors. Both Lee and Symmonds (1972) and Nicholls (1972) mention obesity, smoking, chronic bronchitis, chronic constipation, underlying tissue deficiency and the wearing of tight corsets or constricting garments. All these factors excepting tissue deficiency, will exert their effect through a rise in intra-abdominal pressure, which has been mentioned already as having a most significant role.

By far the most frequently recurring themes, have been the "missed enterocoele" or the inadequately managed enterocoele during primary surgery for prolapse. Once the entity of enterocoele began to achieve recognition, a spate of publications appeared with suggestions as to how the problem should be managed during surgery. Moschcowitz (1912) had described obliteration of the pouch of Douglas to treat rectal prolapse, improving on a purse-string obliteration of the pouch of Douglas proposed by Marion (1909). He used circularly placed sutures of silk, the lowermost suture being placed about one inch above the inferior extremity of the cul-de-sac, with similar sutures, 6—8 in number passed at intervals until practically the entire pouch was obliterated. When sutures reached the region of the supravaginal portion of the cervix and uterine body, he advised anchorage there and furthermore "the ureters and internal iliac vessels should be avoided". The Moschcowitz technique or variant has been the method described in many later reports dealing with abdominal obliteration of the pouch of Douglas to prevent pulsion enterocoele. Frank (1917) in an extensive study of prolapse, suggested oval denudation of the posterior vaginal wall to repair enterocoele and high rectocoele. The peritoneum was pushed as high as possible, opened and obliterated from within, then a purse-string beneath this closure pulled together the uterosacral ligaments and the back of the cervix — "when this stitch is tied, no protrusion of peritoneum or rectum remains". This technique was embellished by Ward (1922) who advised "it is my custom to obliterate the pouch of Douglas by the vaginal or abdominal route, as part of the technique in all cases of operation for prolapse of the uterus". He dissected the sac from below up to the uterosacral ligaments, where it was ligated, cut off, and the uterosacral ligaments united with interrupted linen sutures as close to the rectum as possible.

This then was the key information, namely that an enterocoele must be managed as any other hernia — by the principles of herniotomy and herniorrhaphy. Many authors since these early times, have reinforced this surgical approach. Heaney (1936) gave detailed information about sacrouterine ligament closure; but did not actually mention any specific management of the enterocoele. Meigs (1947) seems first to have mentioned the "overlooked sac" and stressed that the area between the uterosacral ligaments must be inspected during every abdominal hysterectomy and appropriate steps taken to obliterate it. He said, "it is not difficult to see how a small opening between the uterosacral ligaments could be missed; it is hard to visualise; it collapses easily and unless definitely looked for, will be overlooked. There is more interest in the closure of a deep cul-de-sac which is not the source of the hernia." Read (1951) however advised the closure of an abnormally deep or wide pouch of Douglas by excision or circumferentially placed sutures, both procedures being followed by approximation of the uterosacral folds with interrupted sutures. Hiller (1952) advised closing the peritoneum very high posteriorly by putting marked traction on the uterosacral ligaments during vaginal hysterectomy, to minimise recurrence. Later writers Phaneuf (1953), Austin and Damstra (1955), Kinzel (1961), Turner (1961), and Nicholls (1972) have all reinforced the original technique of Frank and Ward and still others have added their own refinements Waters (1955, 1956) stated "there is simply no excuse for vaginal vault prolapse following hysterectomy, for the surgeon should provide adequate support with what tissues he finds by proper choice of procedure and plastic repair of the vaginal walls". To this end he advocated a large wedge shaped resection of the posterior vaginal vault with the base between the utrosacrals and the apex at mid-vagina, together with an adequate lower vaginal reconstruction. This excision altered the vault from cylindrical to conical shape, which supplied a buttress beneath the corrected enterocoele site and removed vault laxity. Symmonds and Pratt (1959) included the Frank-Ward technique together with the vault wedge excision of Waters, and noted that "with these precautions prolapse of the vaginal vault should rarely follow vaginal hysterectomy and repair". Te Linde (1963) suggested that a contributing factor to vault prolapse might be the crushing of the cardinal and uterosacral ligaments, as well as their improper use in vault suspension. In addition, failure to recognize and repair some degree of decensus present at the time of hysterectomy, might lead to a later complete vaginal prolapse. Langmade (1964) seems to have been first to suggest that poor quality tissues associated with the defect were the real problem, and not the failure of surgical technique, for many times he remarked, the uterosacral ligaments were not identifiable as such by even the most expert surgical anatomist, and a suture placed at the site of non-existent uterosacral ligaments offered no support. Shively et al. (1968) recommended closure of the vault after vaginal hysterectomy in a side to side approximation, not the usual inverted "T" closure. The uterosacral and cardinal ligaments sutured together in the midline were attached to the top of the vault posteriorly resulting in a deeper and better supported vagina. Lee and Symmonds (1972) believed many local and general factors favoured recurrence and their prophylaxis meant attention to those key areas which included, proper selection of the operative procedure, proper attention to the cul-de-sac, being aware of deficient post-menopausal tissues, and dealing with obesity, posthysterectomy infection and haematoma. Byron Inmon (1974) endeavoured to minimise post-operative recurrence by attention to two important anatomical principles. Realising the value of both pelvic cellular tissues and levator complex, he attempted the restoration of stretched fascias and ligaments to their normal lengths, as well as repairing striated perineal muscles, so intrapelvic organs could again rest upon the posterior portion of the pubococcygeus muscles. This was the first published attempt to base reconstructive surgery upon anatomical facts, and endeavour to repair specific anatomy which normally supported the genital tract. Clearly the best surgical prophylaxis must be that which corrects normal anatomy so normal function is restored. Feroze (1978) emphasized the point made first by Langmade that despite careful attention to operative technique, enterocoeles will still occur, although maybe some are produced by minimising the degree of high posterior repair in those females to whom a functioning vagina is necessary.

The Surgical Correction of Pulsion Enterocoele

i) Small Pulsion Enterocoele

This variety, the least common must be assumed due to a persistent or recurrent narrow-necked sac following prolapse repair. Many believe a congenital defect of the cul-de-sac or rectovaginal septum is the likely starting point. At a variable time following primary reparative surgery, the patient will notice vague feelings of vaginal pressure, a sensation of something descending the vagina, but usually there are no other symptoms. Examination demonstrates the defect with typical physical signs of enterocoele. It is a slender, often pear-shaped protrusion through the upper posterior vaginal wall, with a narrow neck tapering to a much wider fundus. Until late in its development, marked change in the overlying vaginal epithelium is unusual. Management depends upon size — the larger always need surgical correction, but smaller defects may be reviewed periodically. Surgical correction is straightforward, since the underlying anatomical defects always present with larger examples, are absent. Posterior colpoperineorrhaphy is performed, the posterior vaginal wall being opened either by midline incision, or wedge excision of redundant vaginal epithelium, depending on circumstances. Dissection proceeds to the vaginal vault when the hernial sac is identified and freed from the rectum. Often this separation may be facilitated by placing a sponge forceps with a dampened sponge into the rectum (Ward, 1922). Pushing forward on the forceps, to prolapse the anal canal into the vaginal wound, makes sac delineation above the rectal bulge much easier, faster and safer. The sac is freed as high as possible, until the neck is quite clear of surrounding tissues (Fig. 47). The sac must always be opened to allow inspection of any contents, then it is twisted off firmly, the neck transfixed with "O" Dexon or Vicryl on a Mayo No. 3 roundbodied needle, and the redundancy excised. Using the

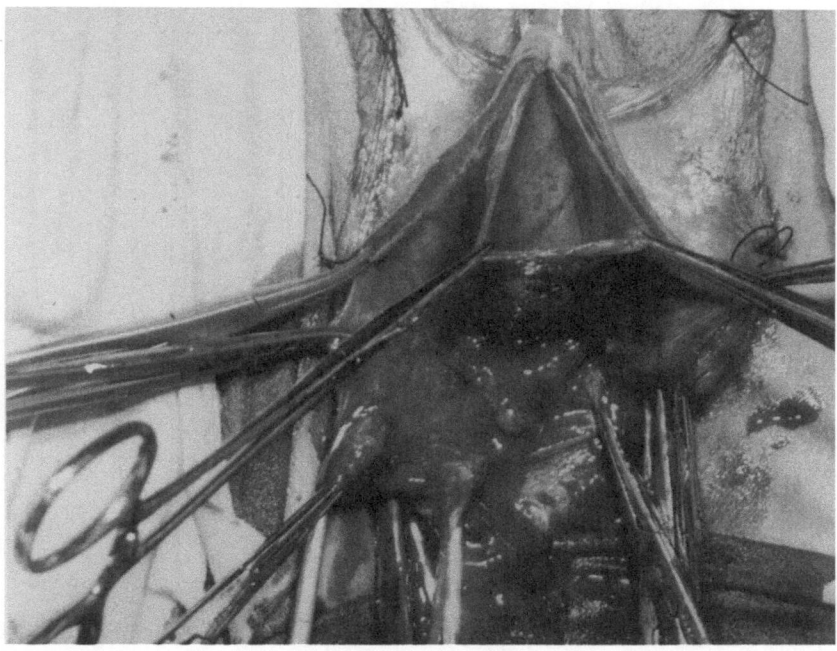

Figure 47. The small enterocoele sac has been isolated from the rectum and opened

transfixion suture, the neck is attached to the epithelium of the vault. This manoeuvre is designed to change direction of the sac and minimise future intra-abdominal pressure thrust. The next step is herniorrhaphy, best achieved by dissecting the rectovaginal septum from the overlying vaginal epithelium, and closing it as a layer over the site of sac excision (Fig. 48). The restored rectovaginal septum acts as a buttress to the excised sac area and anal canal. Finally the vaginal epithelium is closed (with or without excision) using a running locking "O" Dexon or Vicryl suture on a fine cutting edge needle (size 14) which picks up the underlying reconstituted rectovaginal septum. At the lower vagina, near to the fourchette and external anal spincter, one or rarely two sutures are placed to approximate the levator ani. If higher levator sutures are used, not only will they fail to maintain levator approximation, but may produce midvaginal stenosis of variable degree which is better avoided. Posterior vaginal wall closure as described, ensures minimal post-operative haematoma and also a flat surface without stenosis.

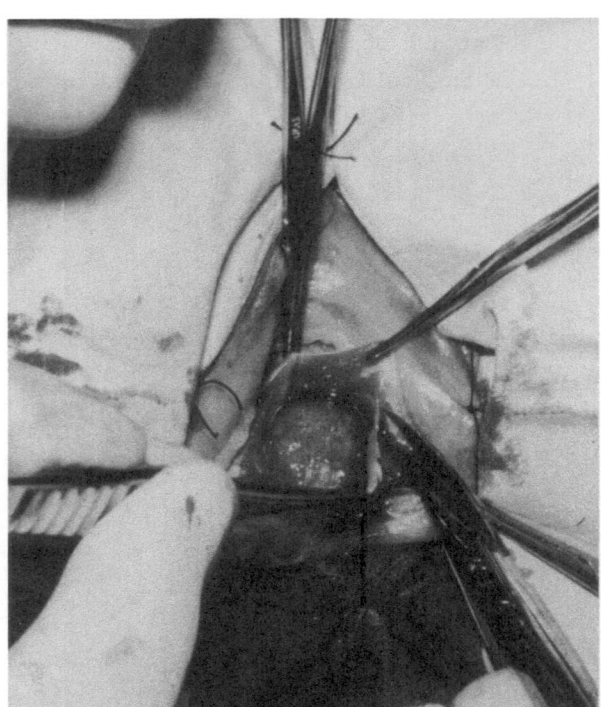

Figure 48 a

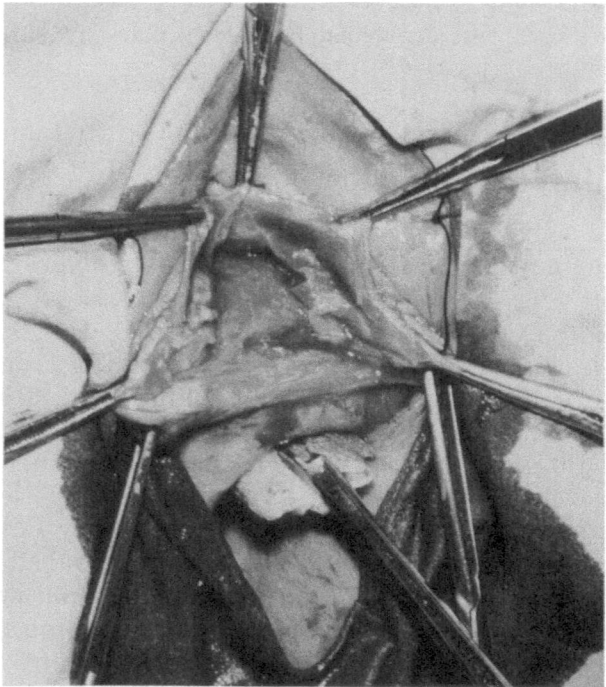

Figure 48 b

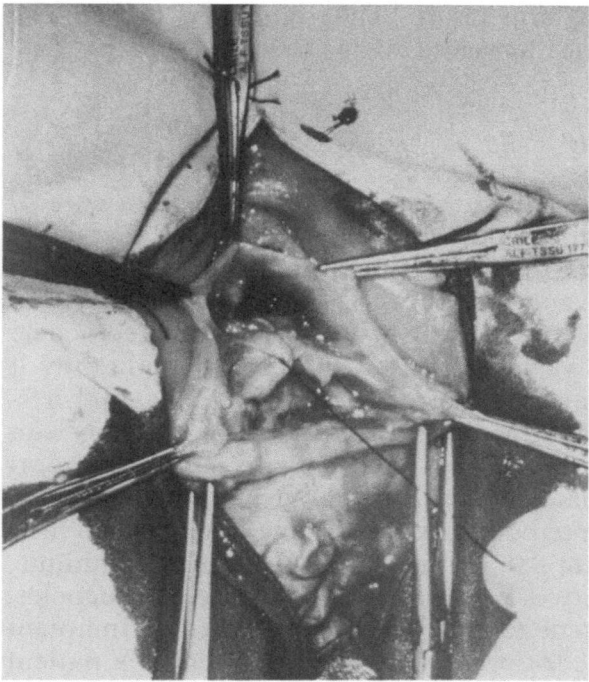

Figure 48 c

Figure 48 a—c. a Sharp dissection separating the fascia of Denonvilliers (rectovaginal septum) from the vaginal epithelium. **b** Completed dissection ready for closure. **c** Closure of the fascial sheet as a separate layer over the closed enterocoele sac

ii) *Medium Pulsion Enterocoele*

The differences between small and medium enterocoele are significant and include a sac with a wider neck, associated vault inversion of variable degree, and commonly an associated rectocoele and/or cystocoele. The differences are due to changes in pelvic cellular tissue and levator complex support, absent with the smaller enterocoele. The medium enterocoele shades gradually into the large, and great care must be taken in deciding which form of surgical correction to advise. Since there is associated damage to key genital tract supporting tissues of variable degree, simple posterior colpoperineorrhyphy with careful attention to the sac cannot always produce the desired longterm result. The significant differences from the small enterocoele, demand a wider choice of therapy.

iii) Large Enterocoele

This problem is merely a further extension of the medium enterocoele with accentuated anatomical defects. The neck of the sac is very wide, reaching out to the general area of the uterosacral ligaments on either side, vault inversion is increased up to total inversion, and because of this a large cystocoele and/or rectocoele are associated, since the vagina is turned inside out. Commonly it develops rapidly following pelvic surgery, particularly vaginal hysterectomy. The problem is caused by a faulty levator complex and pelvic cellular tissues, so even prior to primary surgery the support mechanism was inadequate. If this is true, attempts to prevent a large recurrent pulsion enterocoele, will, in many instances, be ineffectual for it is the patient's tissues rather than surgical technique, which is the fault. Surgery is essential for such large enterocoeles, with the need often urgent to cope with the danger of incipient rupture. There is no place for conservative management in a patient able to undergo surgery, although temporary vaginal packing in hospital might be advantageous in an endeavour to heal over fundal ulceration and minimise post-operative problems of infection.

Surgical Choices

There are four surgical choices available to deal with a large pulsion enterocoele.

  i) Repair by vaginal approach alone.
 ii) Repair by abdominal approach alone.
iii) Colpocleisis.
 iv) Repair by combined abdominal and vaginal approach.

Choice of procedure depends upon many criteria. Most important is the age of the patient and her general condition, the number and variety of previous surgical failures and her wish to continue sexual function. Quite obviously, elderly females in poor general condition should not be subjected to unnecessary major surgery, and particularly is this so when sexual intercourse is no longer required. In these women, the least operative interference which will cure the problem, clearly is the best. Finally, the surgeons choice will be guided by what he believes about the anatomy of genital tract support. He may prefer an empirical symptomatic approach or a specific approach based on factual anatomy of the problem.

Repair by Vaginal Approach Alone

In view of past remarks, it should be obvious that simple posterior colpoperineorrhaphy, even with careful attention to the hernial sac, will, in most instances be quite ineffectual in dealing with a problem of this magnitude. No matter how confidently the surgeon may approach the problem, the vaginal route alone, unless with added features, is doomed because of the nature of the anatomical defect. In particular, the neck of the sac is very wide, there is no worthwhile tissue with which to perform herniorrhaphy, and very wide bites may endanger the ureter (Shaw, 1947), so the sac is dealt with most inadequately, setting the stage for later recurrence. To obviate this problem, extensive skin excision is undertaken, and this unfortunate compromise leads to an unsolved problem, together with a narrowed, often useless vagina (Fig. 49). Langmade et al. (1978) quoted Emil Novak who stated "he had never personally seen a case of vaginal inversion that could not be corrected from below". Berkeley and Bonney (1948) said "they'd not seen a case of inversion that could not be corrected by surgery from below, without shortening the vagina to such an extent that sexual function was impossible". These two divergent opinions were the views of 30 years ago, yet present thoughts about the problem haven't really changed all that much.

Miller (1927) appreciating that vaginal surgery for inverted vagina ended up all too often with a planned or unplanned colpocleisis, devised the following approach: the apex of the inverted vagina was grasped, drawn down and incised transversely below the bladder reflection, and a vertical extension from the midpoint of this incision was made close to the external urethral meatus (Fig. 50). The bladder was mobilised widely, and the paravesical fascia dissected as a distinct layer. After excising vault scar tissue,

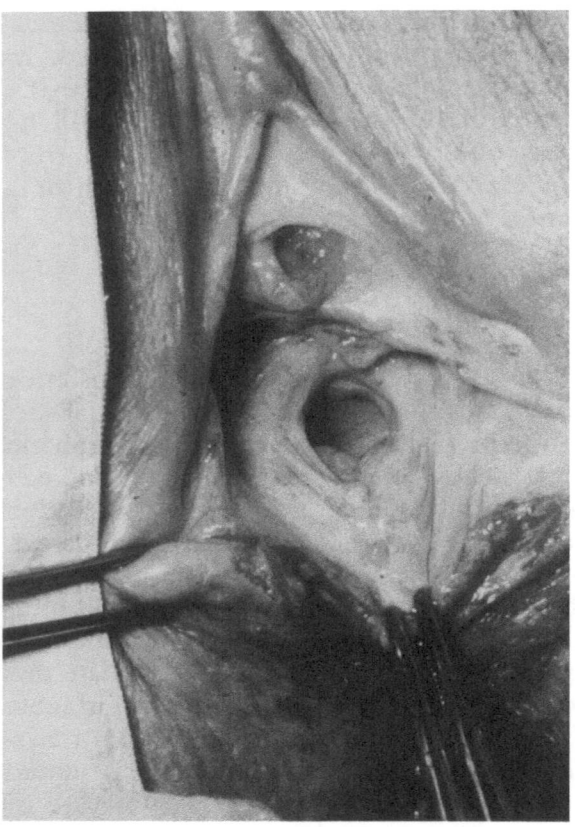

Figure 49. Extreme vaginal stenosis produced by repeated vaginal repairs in a failed endeavour to cure a large enterocoele. Photograph taken following division of the fourchette during reconstruction

the peritoneal cavity was entered and a No. 2 Chromic catgut on a small curved needle guided by the index finger, was passed through peritoneum and underlying fascial and muscular structures at the base of the uterosacral ligament, 1½ inches below the sacral promontory on the right. The procedure was repeated on the left (Fig. 51). The sutures hung free through the peritoneal opening until a fascial overlap beneath the bladder was completed. The free ends of the uterosacral sutures then were passed 2 inches apart through the lower free transverse edge of the overlapped fascial flap. Tying these sutures after peritoneal and vaginal mucosal closure, lifted the vaginal vault and drew it back toward the sacrum (Fig. 52). The end

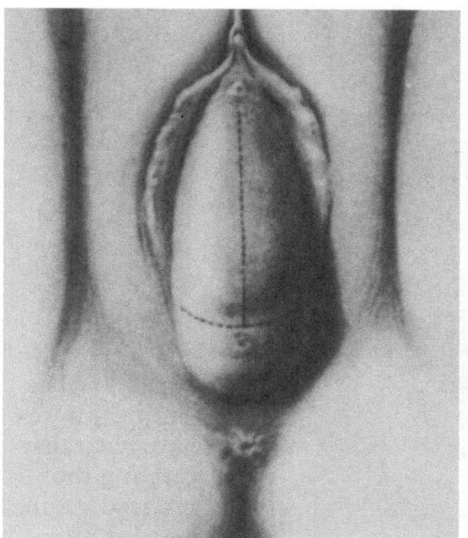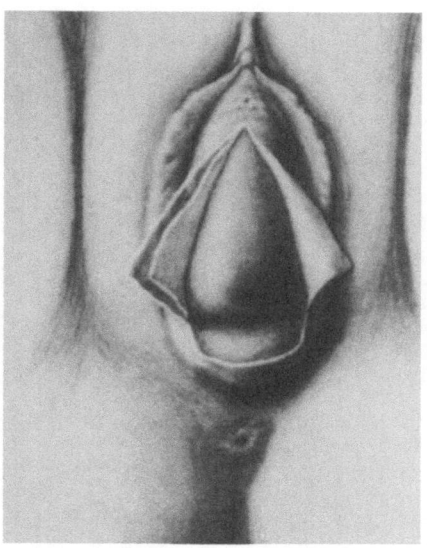

Figure 50. The lines of incision are shown and the dissection of the anterior vaginal wall into its constituent layers. (From Miller)

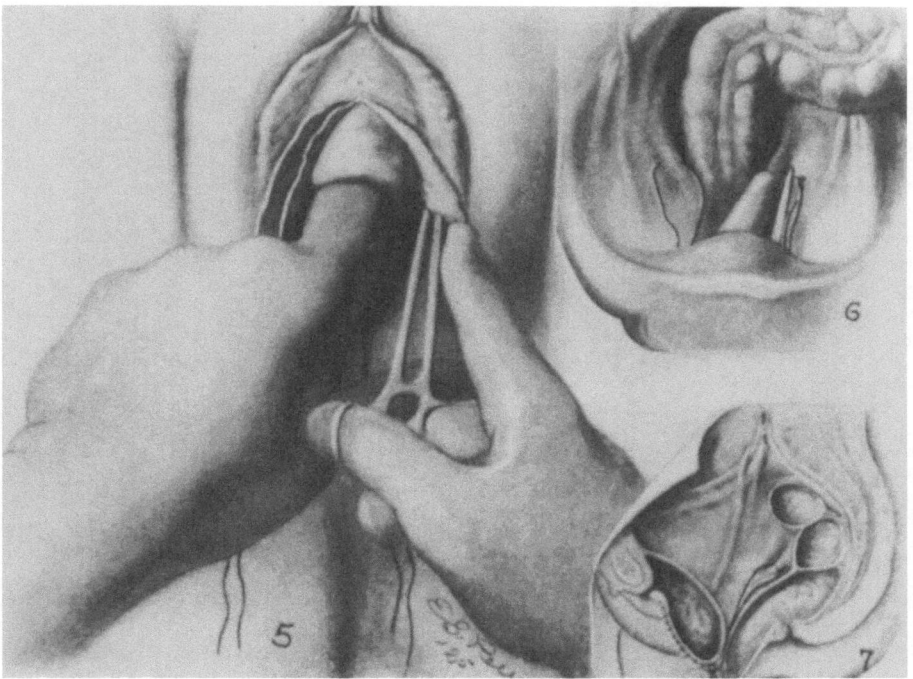

Figure 51. These three diagrams illustrate the blind insertion of the "lifting sutures" into the uterosacral ligament on either side, together with sagittal and coronal views of their position. (From Miller)

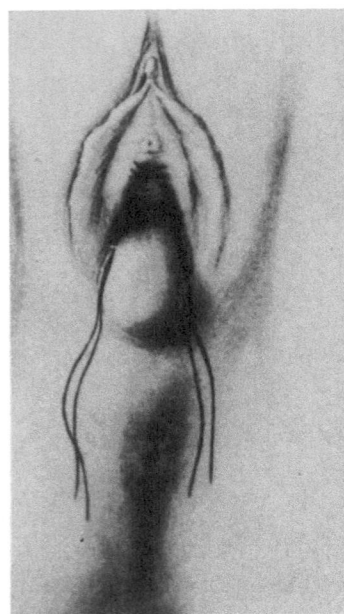
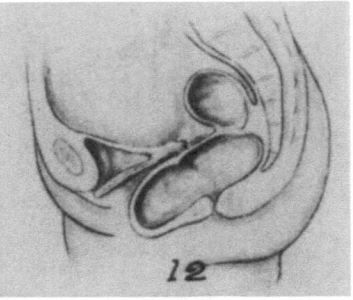
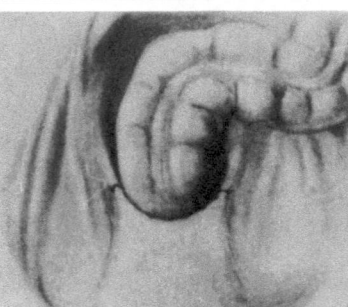

Figure 52. The "lifting sutures" have been tied carrying the inverted vagina high into the pelvis. (From Miller)

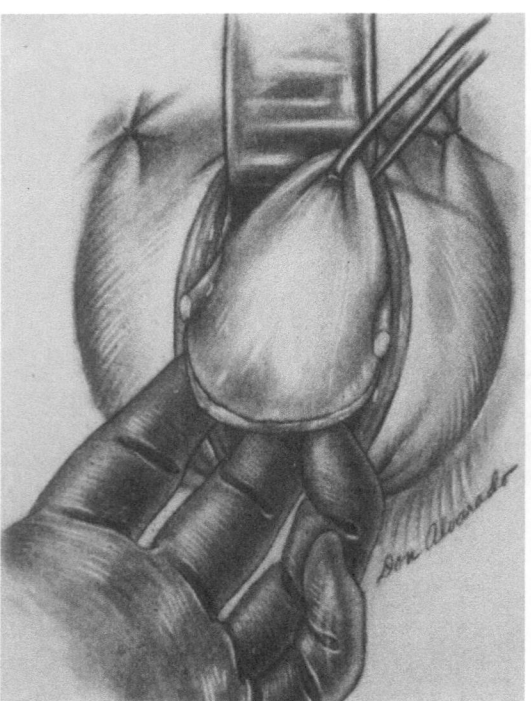
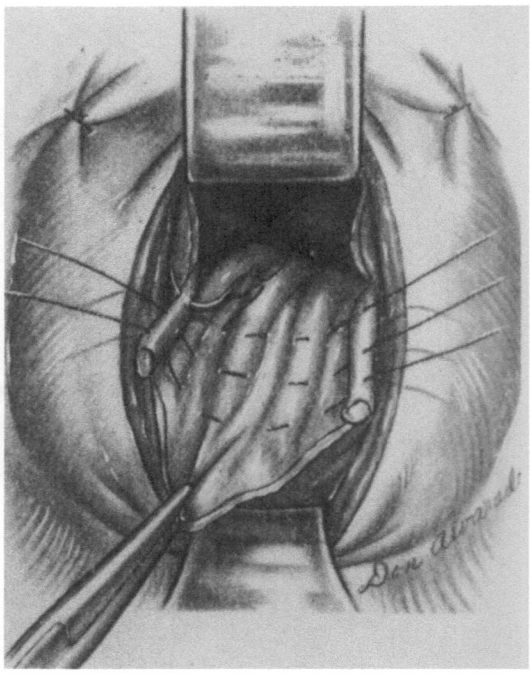

Figure 53 a, b. a Everting the enterocoele sac aids accurate suture placement. Note the ligated ends of the uterosacral ligaments on either side. **b** Non-absorbable sutures pick up the uterosacral ligaments and several bites of redundant pouch of Douglas peritoneum in between. The sutures are placed higher and higher until the entire sac has been picked up. (From McCall)

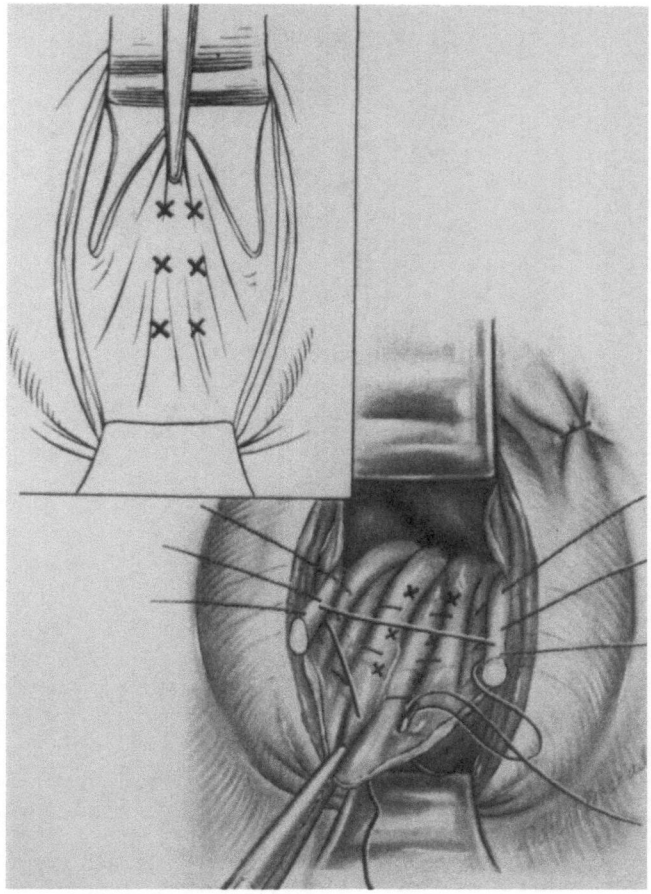

Figure 54. Through and through absorbable sutures are inserted after completing the internal sutures. X marks the entry and exit of each stitch. After passing into the peritoneal cavity from the vagina, each picks up both uterosacral ligaments and passes back to the vagina. These three sutures interdigitate with the internal sutures, the top stitch marking the apex of the reconstructed vagina, and also it incorporates the highest point of the cul de sac relaxation. (From McCall)

result was a functional vagina of normal length and direction and certainly this technique was the precursor of the McCall repair (1957). Both relied on rectification of the pelvic cellular tissue component of the problem, but did nothing to the levator. McCall believed unrepaired high posterior laxity probably was the major

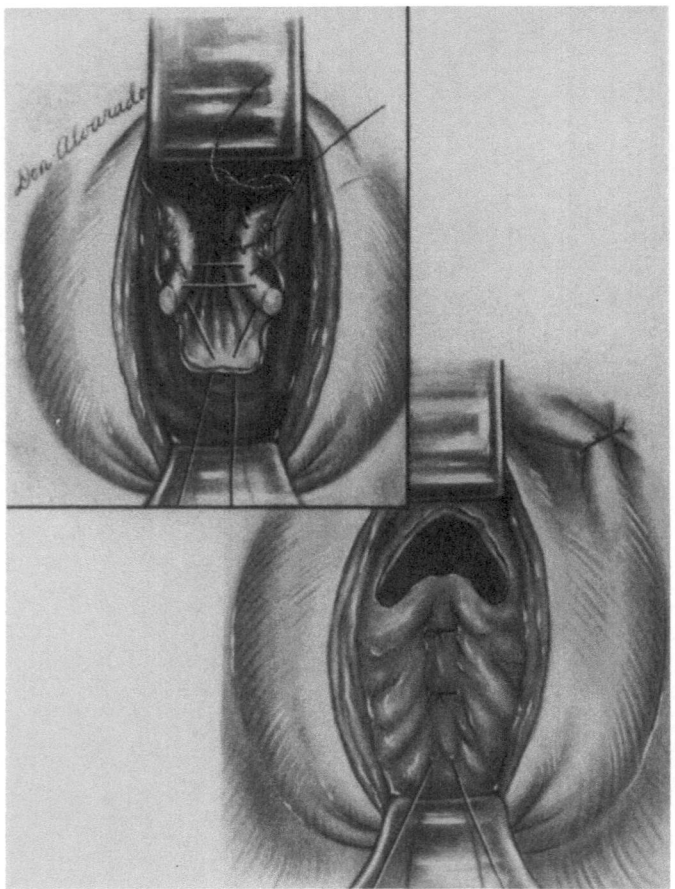

Figure 55 a. First the internal sutures are tied on the peritoneal side followed by tying of the through and through sutures on the vaginal side to obliterate the cul de sac and produce the firm shelf. (From McCall)

cause of recurrent pulsion enterocoele and designed the posterior culdeplasty. Everting the sac, the first intraperitoneal suture picked up the left uterosacral ligament 2 cm above its cut edge and at intervals of 1—2 cm several bites of sac were taken until the right uterosacral ligament was reached and picked up (Fig. 53 a, b). Several similar sutures were placed, picking up all the dependent sac, and with each succeeding suture the relaxed sac was rolled out until the laxity vanished. The next series of sutures began from the

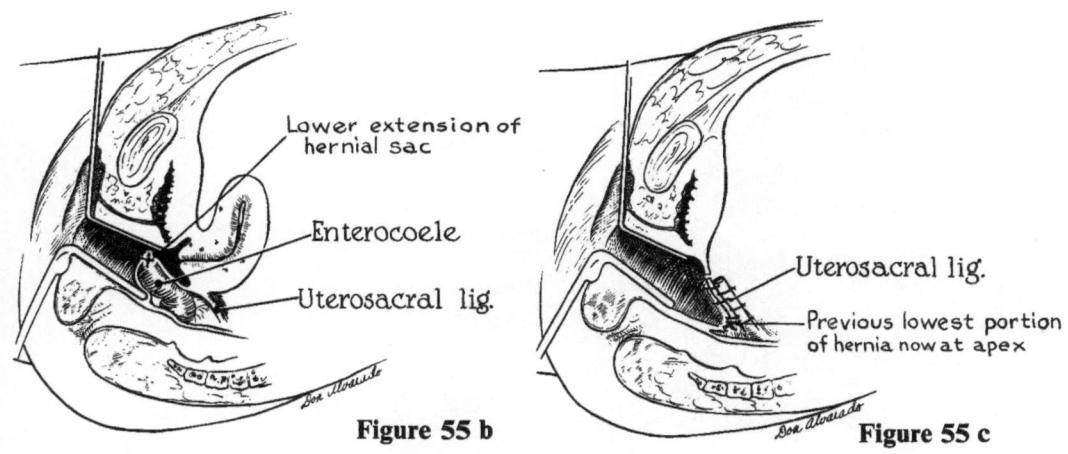

Figure 55 b

Figure 55 c

Figure 55 b, c.
b Line drawing of the enterocoele prior to correction.
c The cul de sac supported by posterior culdeplasty. (From McCall)

vagina just to the right of the midline, 2 cm above the cut edge, entered the peritoneal cavity and picked up both uterosacral ligaments before returning to the vagina, just to the left of the midline at the same level as the entering suture. Usually three such sutures were placed, each higher than the last, lying at intervals between the internal sutures (Fig. 54). The internal sutures were tied obliterating the sac and creating a firm shelf-like structure (Fig. 55 a). With ligation of the external sutures the vaginal wall was pulled into this shelf to fashion a new vault, and because nothing was removed the criticism that most adequate enterocoele repairs shortened the vagina and narrowed the vault was not applicable to posterior culdeplasty (Fig. 55 b, c).

Symmonds and Pratt (1960) extended the McCall technique by dealing with the peritoneal sac at a much higher level: "until the muscularis of the rectosigmoid and rami of the uterosacral ligaments were exposed." They varied the vaginal wall incisions to meet particular circumstances (Fig. 56) enabling decisions about final vaginal depth to be made at the beginning. These incisions were a modification of those suggested by McIntosh Marshall (1953) who performed a very tight vaginal repair with excessive epithelial excision, finishing almost with a total colpectomy. Needless to say he did not have any recurrences of the problem!! Entering the cul-de-sac behind the old vault scar, a finger stretched the anterior wall

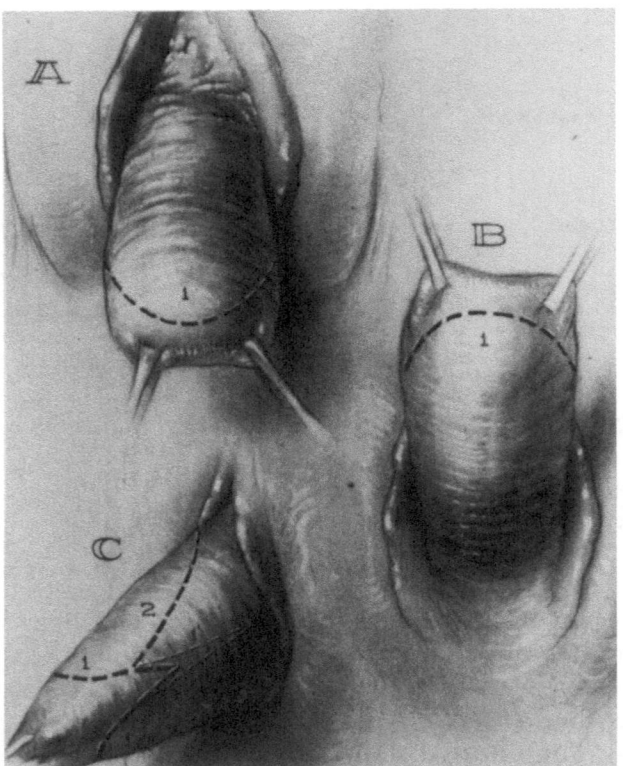

Figure 56. Incisions used by Symmonds and Pratt.
A and *B* are the anterior and posterior elliptical vault incisions. *C* demonstrates how vaginal depth is controlled by the point of union of *A* und *B*. Incision 2 indicates the extent of anterior vaginal wall excision with cystocoele repair. (From Symmonds and Pratt)

of the sac to facilitate bladder mobilisation (Fig. 57). The next step isolated pelvic cellular tissue at each lateral angle of the incision, for they practised block fixation of the uterosacral, cardinal and round ligaments to the lateral angles of the vault, narrowed by wedge excision of the upper posterior vaginal wall (Waters, 1955). Following high sac excision, the uterosacral stumps were pulled together anterior to the rectum and purse-string closure of the peritoneum approximated the rectal and bladder walls closely (Fig. 58). Then the combined stumps were sutured to the lateral angles of the new vault (Fig. 59). The procedure concluded with cystocoele and

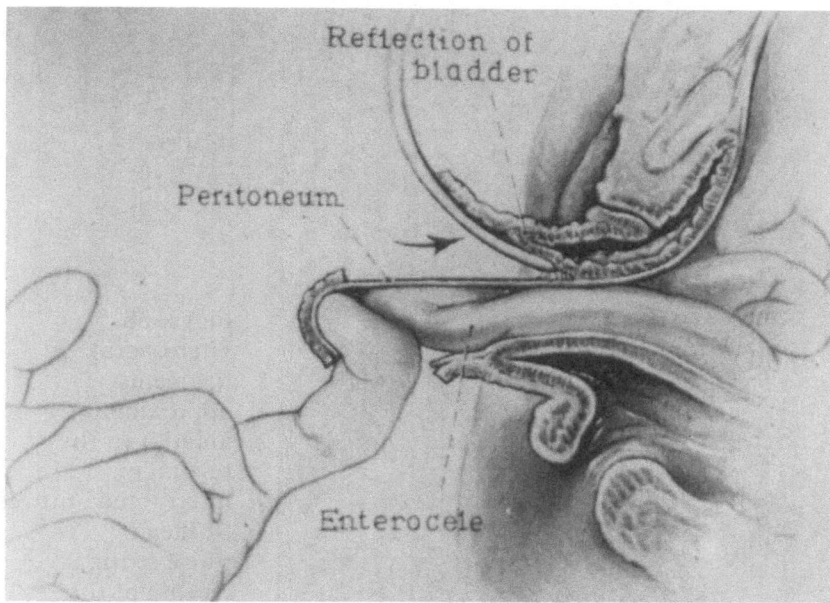

Figure 57. Finger stretches the anterior wall of the sac to facilitate bladder dissection. (From Symmonds and Pratt)

rectocoele repair and produced a well-supported vagina of adequate depth and length, but with a narrowed vault (Fig. 60). They warned of risks to bladder, ureter and rectum. Of 48 vaginal operations reported with adequate follow-up, 7 had recurrent prolapse, 8 had required total vaginectomy, and of the remaining 33 anatomical successes, only 12 reported relatively normal sexual function. Pratt (1966) concluded that no matter how well a secondary vaginal procedure was done, even if the surgeon tried to retain a physiologically useful vagina, the loss of 25—45% of vaginal depth must be anticipated. Beecham and Beecham (1973) commented that such a culdeplasty had a limited practical application, since often the ligaments were atrophic in such females. Randall and Nicholls (1971) believed the technique was satisfactory when the uterosacrals were strong, nevertheless they realised most had defective uterosacrals and proposed vault fixation to the sacrospinous or sacrotuberous ligament in such women. This technique was described first by Zweifel (1892), later by Amreich (1951), Sederl (1958) and Richter (1968). The vault, providing it was of adequate length, could be at-

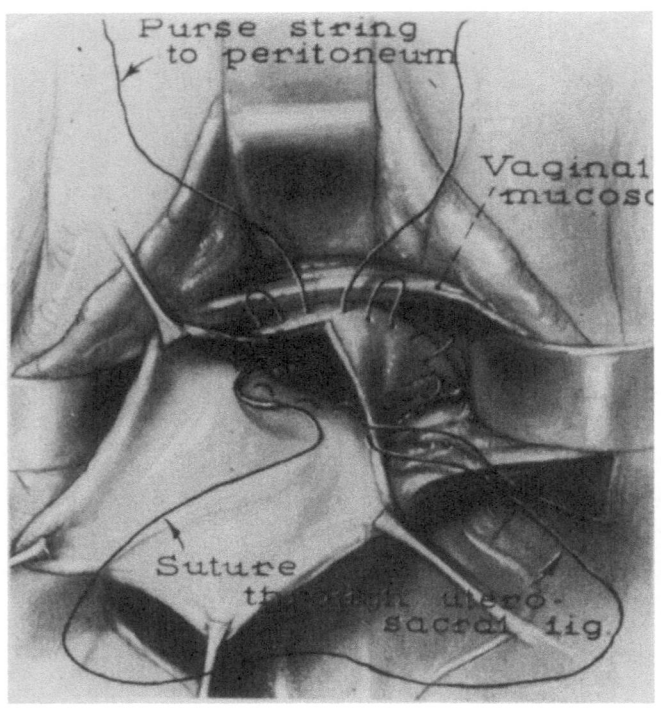

Figure 58.
Uterosacral
ligaments
approximated
anterior to the
rectum by
interrupted sutures
— then a
purse-string
closure of the
peritoneum. (From
Symmonds and
Pratt)

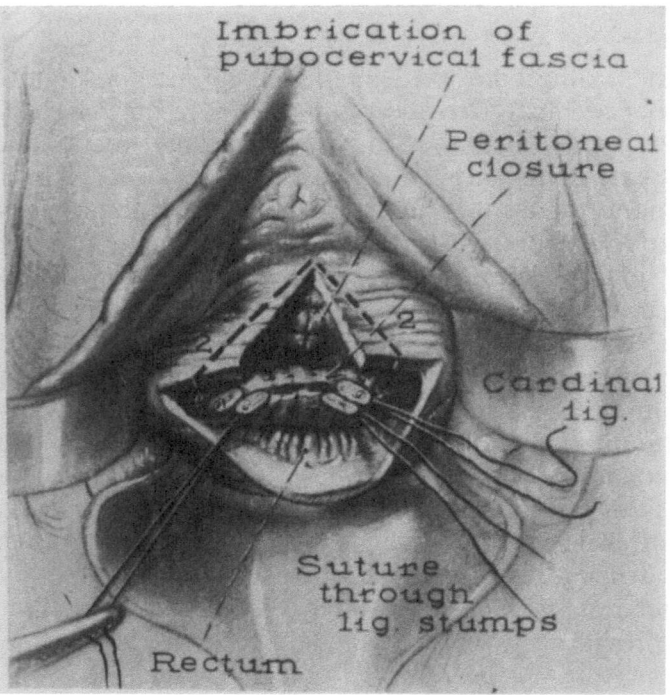

Figure 59. Sac
excision and
closure completed,
the exteriorised
ligament stumps
are secured to the
new vault angles
and then the
cystocoele is
repaired. (From
Symmonds and
Pratt)

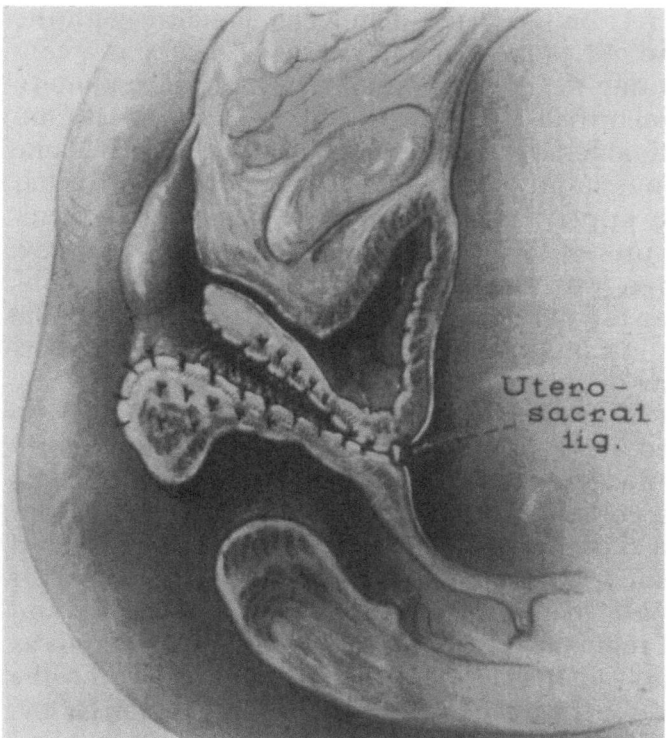

Utero-
sacral
lig.

Figure 60. The end result showing a vagina of adequate length and diameter, but with some coning at the vault. (From Symmonds and Pratt)

tached transvaginally to the sacrospinous ligament, the suture being placed blindly but guided by the index finger which identified the ischial spine. This technique restored the horizontal axis of the vagina. Birnbaum (1973) drew attention to the attendant risks of damage to the pudendal vessels and sciatic nerve with this technique.

Inmon (1974) seems to have been first in appreciating that both levator and pelvic cellular tissue defects were at the root of the problem and devised a vaginal technique to restore their support roles. He realised the cardinal ligaments acted to hold the genital tract in place against strong forces endeavouring to displace it from the correct position over the levator plate and said "specifically stretched fascias and ligaments must be restored to normal lengths and striated perineal muscles must be repaired so that the intrapelvic organs again rest on the plate". The technique dealt with the sac appropriately and closed the rectovaginal septal tissues as a continuous layer. Reflecting the epithelium laterally the cardinal-utero-sacral bundle was identified almost to the lateral pelvic wall, and sutures drew these ligamentous bundles together until they became tight cords. Additional sutures were placed to achieve even further shortening, then the upper margin of the previously closed recto-vaginal fascia was sutured to the shortened ligamentous complex. Perineal muscle repair was essential and needed to be meticulous and adequate so that the perineal body would be the length of the urethra, for then the intrapelvic organs would rest on the plate. Possibly Inmon's perineal repair produced tensing of the plate by approximating the crural margins anterior to the anal canal. Symmonds (1980) devised a more efficient method of isolating the utero-sacral ligament remnants. When the prolapsed vault was opened, the peritoneum was entered anteriorly and posteriorly, the entries being separated by a skin bridge at the site of the vault scar. Lateral vaginal skin was pushed as high as possible using the skin bridge for traction, the ureter was identified by palpation on either side and then the uterosacral remnant was clamped with a Heaney clamp as high as possible. Each ligament was transfixed and held, then the skin bridge removed. Wedge excision of vaginal epithelium at the vault was performed and left attached inferiorly by its apex, upon which the Auvard speculum rested. The peritoneum was stripped from the lower rectum until it could be stripped no further and classical McCall sutures were inserted in the vault. The posterior vaginal wall was repaired in one layer with interrupted sutures, which picked up skin, pararectal tissues and skin, similar in intent to the vault McCall sutures. Near to the perineum, the levator crura were exposed in the pararectal space and sutures passed through skin, crus and pararectal fascia of one side then the other, to exit through skin in series with the upper posterior vaginal wall sutures. Numerous small sutures approximated the perineal muscles. So this may be regarded as the definitive vaginal technique for a large pulsion enterocoele, combining the best of Inmon and McCall with carefully considered additions by Symmonds. However, although presently the best available vaginal technique, unless performed meticulously avoiding the many anatomical pitfalls, the end result will be less than good with recurrence likely. No matter how carefully the procedure is done some vaginal shortening is inevitable.

Repair by Abdominal Approach Alone

As early as 1927, gynaecologists had considered the abdominal route to cope with the difficult problem of large pulsion enterocoele, spurred on by two facts — first, a realisation of the inadequacies of the vaginal approach alone, and second, the cure rate for rectal prolapse achieved by the Moschcowitz procedure.

Fraenkel (1927) and Jarcho (1928) described ventrofixation of the vagina as a method of curing genital prolapse (Fig. 61), which was safe, simple, and effective, and recurrence was due they believed, to faulty technique. No patient numbers were mentioned, minor strangury persisted for a few days only and no recurrences were recorded.

Ward (1929) believed that closure of the cul-de-sac by the Moschcowitz technique, caused the viscera to be thrown forward onto the bladder, pubic symphysis and anterior abdominal wall when the patient was erect, and advocated obliteration of the cul-de-sac as an important part of his surgical technique in all cases of prolapse. Brady (1936) considered prolapse after panhysterectomy to be a far more difficult situation to correct than the original prolapse, and some gynaecologists believed there was no satisfactory procedure available. Brady reported an operation on one patient only, which lifted the vaginal vault by 3 braided silk sutures passed through the peritoneum medial to the rectus muscles and out through the anterior sheath to be tied, so fixing the vagina to the anterior abdominal wall. Review at nine months was satisfactory.

So began the great empirical onslaught lifting the vaginal vault and fixing it to something, which has persisted to this day. Few who have employed these techniques ever seemed concerned with such an unanatomical approach and fewer still were interested in this gross departure from the normal anatomy of vaginal support. The fact that the normal vagina was supported in a very different way from the end result of such procedures didn't worry the perpetrators at all, and they blamed failures on technical errors. Succeeding papers in addition to becoming more ingenious, became obsessed with operative technique with little or no attention paid to specific anatomical reconstruction. Later technical reports commonly failed to acknowledge the fact that the procedure had been described previously.

Grant Ward (1937) reduplicated the round ligaments using ox

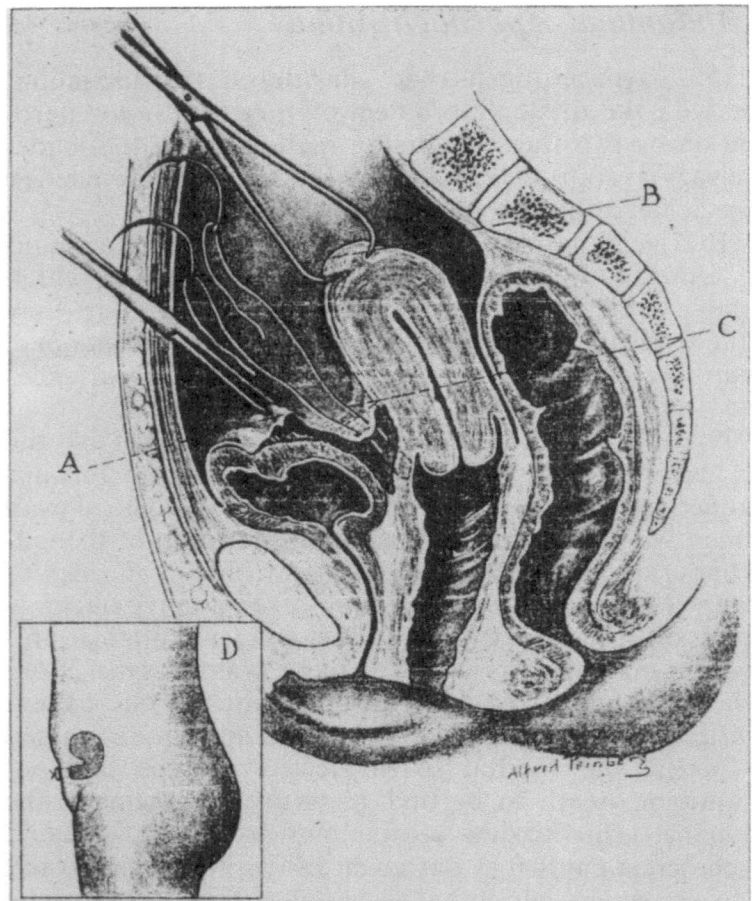

Figure 61. Jarcho's technique of vaginal ventrofixation.
A Allis forceps on the vesico-vaginal peritoneal fold. *B* Vulsellum grasping the uterine fundus. *C* Sutures passed through the vaginal vault and peritoneum. *D* Uterine position after completing the procedure. (From Jarcho)

fascia lata knowing of its use in the repair of other herniae. The fascia was passed from either angle of the vaginal vault, following the course of the round ligament extraperitoneally to be fixed on the anterior surface of the posterior rectus sheath. So the vault was supported by these new round ligaments, despite the fact that under normal conditions round ligaments played no part in genital tract support. Fletcher (1947) in his procedure of abdominal colpocystopexy added the Moschcowitz procedure to vault suspension and achieved the result by what he termed "a crossed suspender support". Following pouch of Douglas obliteration, only the vagina above the uterosacral ligaments was mobile and required fixation. A long vagina was stabilised by ventrofixation; but the short was managed by two crossed fascial strips cut from the anterior rectus sheath, with their base about 6 cm above the pubis. The strip was passed through the rectus muscle and peritoneum, down to the lateral limits of the vaginal cuff on the opposite side, where it was fixed. The strip had to be long enough to allow proper bladder filling. He reported a short follow-up on 7 patients. Shaw (1947) added a minor variant to earlier techniques by cutting aponeurotic strips from both internal and external oblique muscles through a Pfannenstiel incision and then passing them down along the course of the round ligaments, and Guiou (1949) used a similar procedure.

Arthure and Savage (1957) suggested posterior vault fixation, a new approach, which they termed "sacral hysteropexy". This procedure fixed the vaginal vault to the intervertebral disc between the 5th lumbar and 1st sacral vertebra, the lateral spaces being made extraperitoneal. Although they reported only 5 failures with 48 patients in a 5 year period and a less anatomical approach would be difficult to imagine, nevertheless it did return the vaginal vault over the levator plate; but an ineffectual levator plate. Falk (1960) believed pouch of Douglas obliteration was essential and announced his enthusiasm for sacral hysteropexy. Embrey (1961) realised that a major fault with ventrosuspension was the risk of enterocoele, since in this incorrect anatomical position the posterior vaginal wall now bore the full brunt of intra-abdominal pressure.

The Burch procedure of urethrovaginal fixation to Cooper's ligament in the management of recurrent stress incontinence of urine was reported in 1961, and the chief complication mentioned was enterocoele which occurred four times early on in the development of the technique. Later cases included the Moschcowitz procedure believing enterocoele development would no longer be a major problem. Accordingly Embrey favoured posterior fixation and modified the Arthure: Savage procedure using a fascial sling between the vaginal vault and sacrum. Three of his first 6 cases recurred, but in the succeeding 12 the result was satisfactory. Lane (1962) added lower abdominal pain and recurrence of prolapse when the patient sat, to the difficulties of ventrofixation and suggested retrofixation by synthetic material, initially to a stainless steel pin driven into the sacrum, later modified to the fixing of synthetic material to the anterior longitudinal ligament. The 20 cases he reported had only a short follow-up, with some early recurrences.

Langmade (1964) noted current problems with vault suspension methods and laid down criteria for success, in particular that strong separate autogenous tissues should be used for the supports, with vault traction forces directed laterally as in normal support. A lax anterior abdominal wall was unsatisfactory for holding up the vault and any method chosen should not require additional incisions, or be followed by incisional hernia. It should be performed easily with low morbidity and Langmade's solution gained from cadaver dissections was to use Astley Cooper's ligament after detaching it from the inner pubic ramus.

Ferguson (1964) returned to ventrofixation using Marlex mesh introduced along the course of the round ligament and supported the procedure with one case. Bremer (1965) made a strong plea for the abdominal approach as the "only remaining one" since the results of vaginal correction were so poor in terms of scarring and recurrence, and his contribution to ventrofixation was the use of synthetics such as Dacron aortic bifurcation graft inverted and used as the Marlex mesh described previously by Ferguson. Welsh (1967) and Dastur et al (1967) described synthetic slings to correct procidentia — Welsh reduplicated the round ligaments and the Shirodkar sling used by Dastur et al., reduplicated the uterosacral ligaments. Soichet (1969) used silastic silicone rubber to suspend the vagina from the lumbosacral cartilage. Richardson and Williams (1969) preferred mersilene tape but noted that urinary problems could occur if it was attached too far down the anterior vaginal wall. Attachment too far down the posterior wall might allow the anterior vaginal wall to sag and the cystocoele to bulge. Thursz (1970) returned to ventrofixation with synthetic tape but Freedman and Meltzer (1970) used collagen mesh to substitute for the uterosacral, cardinal and round ligaments. The anterior and posterior vaginal walls were invested with sheets of mesh 5 × 3 cm, then mesh strips in substitution for the ligaments were sutured to the angles of the vault. The round ligament strip was anchored antrolaterally to the tendon of the rectus abdominis on the superior aspect of the pubic bone, the cardinal to the ileopectineal crest and the uterosacral to the aponeurotic insertion of the coccygeus on the front of the sacrum, and finally the whole prosthesis was located extraperitoneally. Applied to two patients with success, this technique was the first real attempt by the abdominal route to reduplicate pelvic cellular tissue anatomy, but the levator complex was ignored completely.

Lee and Symmonds (1971) reviewed various techniques used to correct vault inversion and suggested the abdominal approach for severe or recurrent vault inversion was best, because of dissatisfaction with accepted methods of vaginal repair. They emphasized the importance of adding a Moschcowitz type procedure to vault suspension, to avoid recurrent enterocoele. Birnbaum (1973) despite quoting Ball who had said "the illogicality of attempting to correct this condition from the abdominal route was apparent to anyone with the simplest knowledge of the mechanics of the female pelvic floor" nevertheless believed the abdominal approach had major advantages. Existing vaginal calibre and depth could be retained, and the surgeon could identify vault, bladder, rectum and ureters with certainty. The major problem with available operations was anterior rotation of the vaginal axis to assume a position perpendicular to and almost directly over the levator hiatus, at the point where the vagina perforated the levator sling and urogenital diaphragm. He appreciated the need to fix the vaginal vault over the levator plate, and employed Teflon mesh sited extraperitoneally to fix the vault low down on the sacrum. He termed the technique "sacral colpopexy", which corrected vault prolapse but not cystocoele or rectocoele which needed additional surgery. He reported on 9 patients. As with the Arthure: Savage sacral hysteropexy, one might well ponder the use of retrofixation without correction of an ineffectual levator plate.

Beecham and Beecham (1973) concerned that the McCall culdeplasty had limitations, and by the low but persistent rate of foreign body reaction and infection in dorsal vault fixation techniques using synthetic materials, put forward yet another version of ventrosuspension. Using fascia lata obtained with a Masson stripper, they anchored the apex and upper posterior third of the vaginal vault to the anterior rectus sheath 3 cm above the pubis. The strip lay in a tunnel between bladder and peritoneum, and success was claimed in 12 patients. Tomlinson and Alexander (1974) resurrected the Bremer operation using a Dacron aortic bifurcation graft prosthesis. They commented on the pain-free coughing allowed by the elasticity of the prosthesis.

Sivasuriya (1974) sutured the round ligaments to the vault angles in an attempted revival of the principle of the Grant Ward technique whilst Rust et al. (1975) rediscribed the Arthure: Savage procedure, and Yates (1975) enthused over the "sacro-colpopexy" identical to that of Birnbaum. Inmon and Bledsoe (1975) reporting genital prolapse in a patient after hemipelvectomy, stated principles which must be observed for success in vault inversion surgery. The vaginal cuff must be fixed at or near its original position, fascial and ligamentous laxity must be corrected and adequate perineal muscle repair accomplished, so intrapelvic organs rested on the levator plate.

Todd (1977) returned to sacral fixation using a loop of synthetic mesh, the ends of which were attached to the sacral promontory and the mid portion to the vault. The inferior free edge was attached to the lateral peritoneum and the idea was to reconstitute the uterosacral ligaments. Lin (1978) sutured the stretched vagina by a series of 8—10 concentric purse-string "O" silk sutures to the sacrum and Langmade et al. (1978) noted some 43 procedures had been devised through the years for this problem indicating the poor success rate, yet again came out in favour of Astley Cooper's ligament suspension which Langmade had reported 18 years before. Despite their enthusiasm, 15% of their 63 cases recurred. Kaskarelis (1978) again described the principle of Brady's operation using 3 silk sutures on either side from the vault passing to the front of the rectus sheath and tied firmly.

From 1970 to 1976 many papers from European clinics reported on their experience with vault suspension by various methods. Wyka (1970) sutured the vault to the sacral promontory as did Von Kraatz (1972) and Von Grunberger (1976). From Czechoslovakia (1973) came a report on 5 cases using Cooper's ligament and from Paris (1974) the use of sacral fixation.

Feldman and Birnbaum (1979) reported a further series of Teflon sacral colpopexy involving 21 patients with good results up to 4 years.

Cowan and Morgan (1980) used mersilene mesh initially and proline mesh in later cases. In a series of 39 patients they recorded one recurrence. Lansman (1984) reported a series of 8 patients in whom sacral colpopexy was achieved by the use of a dura mater graft. Follow-up was short term only.

Over a similar time interval abdominal attempts to rectify rectal prolapse, not surprisingly, have shown many similarities to the surgery of vaginal vault inversion. Jeannel (1896) described anterior abdominal wall and pelvic brim fixation of the mobilised rectum and a similar procedure, the Pemberton-Stalker operation was published in 1939, but as with the abdominal repair of pulsion enterocoele, longer follow-up revealed many recurrences (17 of 52).

The Wells (1962) and Ripstein (1963) operations both superceded other procedures, for each endeavoured to repair the levator defect and replace the prolapsed rectum over the levator plate by fixing the rectum in the sacral hollow with synthetic material. In 1952, Lahaut had suggested implanting the mobilised rectosigmoid in the posterior rectus sheath to avoid the use of foreign materials, but other problems — incisional hernia and faecal fistula — were produced. Dendy Moore (1977) to avoid synthetic materials used ventrofixation to the anterior abdominal wall in 42 patients with good results apart from a lower abdominal bulge and Graham et al. (1984) promoted sacral fixation to avoid foreign materials. Their 23 patients showed good longterm benefits.

The overiding picture of the abdominal approach has been dissatisfaction with available procedures. Additionally and most importantly, these techniques are certainly not free from serious complications. Ventrofixation may produce a degree of bladder dysfunction, abdominal wall tenderness and without cul-de-sac obliteration, leave the way open for enterocoele development. Retrofixation has resulted in more serious complications. Sutton et al. (1981) encountered serious venous bleeding from presacral veins and haemostasis was a great problem. Any method of sacral fixation is liable to this potentially hazardous complication. Both ventro and retrofixation are prone to recurrence varying with differing methods, with ileus and small bowel obstruction being reported in most series. Synthetic materials can be rejected, become infected leading to persistent sinus formation and disintegrate or pull out from the tissues with disastrous results. Fascial strips, often from the abdominal wall leave areas of weakness, and a poor quality abdominal wall after ventrofixation can allow prolapse to recur when the abdominal wall relaxes.

Fixing the vault anteriorly, laterally and posteriorly have been tried and retried, so obviously the longterm result has been found wanting, or one procedure now would be well established, and the others discarded. This has not happened and is unlikely, for little or no consideration has been given in any of these purely empirical techniques, to the twin underlying defects of the levator complex and pelvic cellular tissues. Admittedly, those espousing retrofixation beginning with Arthure and Savage, and the attempt by Freedman and Meltzer to reconstitute the pelvic cellular tissues were steps in the right direction; but success was not to be achieved longterm until and unless both defects received attention.

Although many types of vault fixation have been described through the years, with variable results, this empirical approach cannot be the correct way to deal with the large pulsion enterocoele and the right way has got to be attempts to reconstitute the normal supporting anatomy.

Colpocleisis

First performed in 1867 and reported in 1881 by Neugebauer, colpocleisis has undergone many periods of acceptance and rejection as a method of dealing with prolapse. Known more usually as the Neugebauer - Le Fort or even the Le Fort after the French gynaecologist published his report in 1877, over the years numerous case reports have appeared generally favouring the procedure in a limited group of patients, providing certain technicalities were observed. The operation provides great symptomatic relief in a difficult situation, often in a poor risk surgical patient.

Falk and Kaufmann (1955) reported their experiences with 100 patients stating that most suitable was the elderly female with complete vaginal eversion and a poor risk for surgery, for it was a comparatively short procedure requiring only light anaesthesia, but obviously the patient and her husband must understand that intercourse could no longer be possible afterwards. Two problems encountered after colpocleisis were poor healing of opposed vaginal tissues and the occurrence of post-operative stress incontinence of urine, due it was believed to traction on the anterior vaginal wall, disturbing upper urethral mechanics.

The standard procedure was applied to procidentia with the uterus still present so drainage tracts to permit the escape uf uterine secretions were left on either side. Commencing with dilatation and curettage, rectangular areas of vaginal epithelium were removed from the anterior and posterior vaginal walls and the prolapse reduced by suturing the denuded areas together, commencing near the external os. When completed, the uterus opened into a narrowed transverse canal which communicated with the lateral canals on either side. Too much excision of anterior vaginal wall tissue beneath the urethra must not occur; but an exact spot was difficult to define. Hanson and Keetel (1969) discussed 288 patients in whom 20 developed stress incontinence and 13 a recurrence of the prolapse — in 3 there was complete breakdown but cured by a repeat Le Fort procedure. They did not believe the risk of undetected endometrial carcinoma was real, because of the drainage canals.

Diddle (1970) reported 3 patients in whom a modified Le Fort operation had corrected complete vault inversion following hysterectomy. He excised vaginal epithelium from each lateral side leaving intact a midline strip on both anterior and posterior walls, then the raw lateral surfaces were approximated to avoid pulling on the bladder floor. A perineorrhaphy completed the surgery. All were cured and none reported stress incontinence.

Ridley (1972) pointed out the select place of colpocleisis in the management of prolapse, whilst detailing its disadvantages. He criticised the various modifications of colpocleisis "to increase its scope" (Goodall and Power, 1937) for procedures less than complete colpocleisis which advocated partial occlusion of only the upper two-thirds of the vagina, had an increased incidence of failure. He described his experience with 58 operations performed for complete vaginal prolapse either primary or recurrent. Vaginal hysterectomy and repair had largely replaced the Le Fort operation in later years as anaesthesia etc., had improved and he believed the uterus should be removed if possible because of the cancer risk or even a troublesome discharge. He noted 5 cases developed stress incontinence and blamed a downward displacement of the bladder with distortion of the posterior urethrovesical angle, so advocated vaginal occlusion only above this area. In 3 of his patients, the prolapse had recurred in a short time. Rust et al. (1976) regarded colpocleisis almost as an historical procedure, because of the other techniques that avoided the failure rates, urinary incontinence and loss of sexual function. However Ardekany and Rafee (1978) believed colpocleisis was the procedure of choice in the management of procidentia in post-menopausal females. They described a T-shaped anterior and posterior vaginal wall skin excision beginning 1.5 cm below the external urethral meatus and ceasing 2 cm from the external os. The posterior excision was completed by a perineorrhaphy excision. The modification in their technique was minimal excision so much less traction on the bladder and urethra resulted. Fifteen cases were reported and the 11 traced patients were cured. Goldman et al. (1981) discussed 118 patients. They limited the anterior rectangular excision to avoid urethral traction and performed a high posterior perineorrhaphy to give good posterior support. They recorded only 3 recurrences and no longterm urinary problems. One patient required hysterectomy for bleeding. Jones (1981) reviewing the procedure, concluded that it was most useful following failure to cure procidentia, due not to the surgeon but to tissues which had no substance.

The Place of Colpocleisis in the Correction of Large Pulsion Enterocoele

Nowadays there are very few patients with procidentia unable to tolerate vaginal hysterectomy and a tight vaginal repair, for this is the ideal method to deal with the problem. Colpocleisis is better avoided when the uterus is present, its place "par excellence" being the elderly female with recurrence of pulsion enterocoele following pelvic surgery, in whom there is no requirement to preserve sexual function. With good pre-operative preparation and expert anaesthesia there is minimal upset to the patient. The original Neugebauer - Le Fort is no longer necessary because when the procedure has been modified to lessen the risk of urinary complications, the risk of failure and prolapse recurrence has increased. The tissues in such patients are very poor quality so every effort must be made to minimise recurrence.

Technique

Pre-operative Dienoestrol cream and Acijel used alternately prepare the vaginal environment adequately for surgery. With the patient in lithotomy position the labia are stitched back and the extent of the vaginal inversion inspected. It is usual for at least the lower part of the anterior vaginal wall to be undisturbed, and often the inversion is mainly posterior vaginal wall stopping at the vault scar of the previous hysterectomy. The skin bulge is picked up with 3 Allis forceps — top, middle and bottom, and drawn down to appreciate the full extent of the bulge and adjustments to the siting of the clamps are

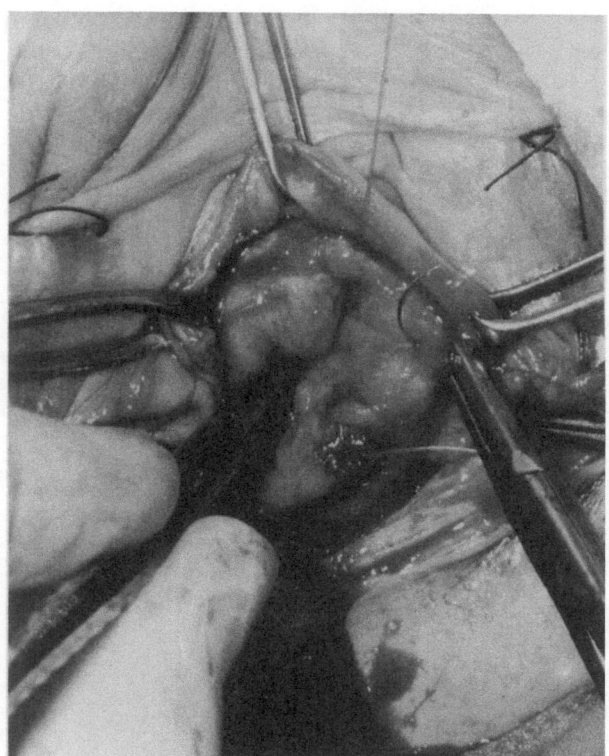

Figure 62. Wide denudation of vaginal epithelium completed, a series of concentric purse-string sutures begins

made. It is most important that all redundant epithelium is removed (Fig. 62). When denudation is complete, gradually the enterocoele sac is reduced by a series of concentric 2/0 chromic catgut purse-string sutures, until a flat surface presents (Fig. 63 a, b). There is no benefit at all in opening the sac during this procedure. At this point, the posterior colpoperineorrhaphy begins with wide excision of the fourchette between Allis forceps, and the posterior vaginal wall skin is excised to the enterocoele area. The rectovaginal septum is freed from the overlying vaginal skin on either side and closed with a running suture of "O" Vicryl, then a small ovoid of mersilene mesh is fitted over the flat enterocoele area and the closed recto-vaginal septum, and anchored by a series of 2/0 chromic catgut sutures to the deep aspect of the overlying skin (Fig. 64). The vaginal skin is closed with a running locking suture of 2/0 Vicryl in

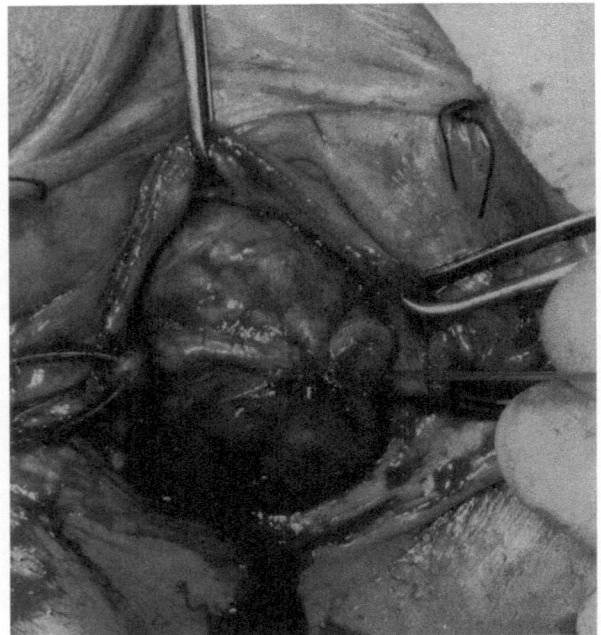

Figure 63 a, b. a Gradual reduction of the enterocoele bulge by the series of inverting purse-string sutures. **b** The flat surface which results when the bulge is reduced completely

Figure 63 a

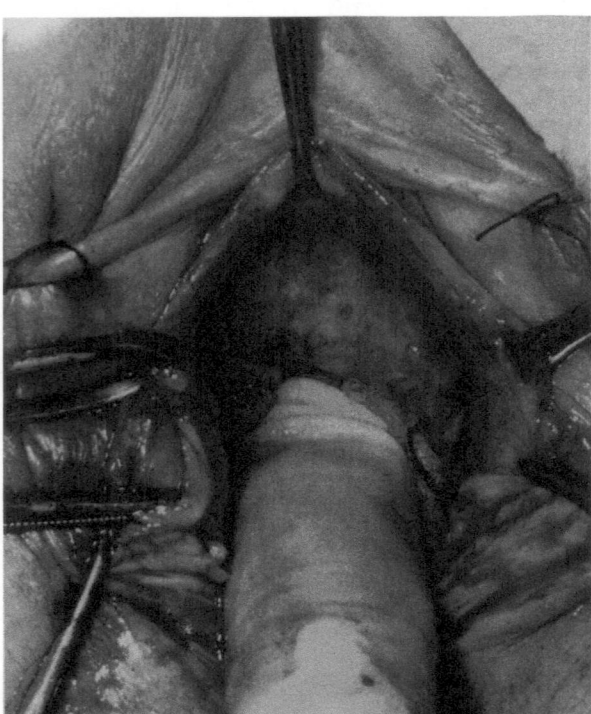

Figure 63 b

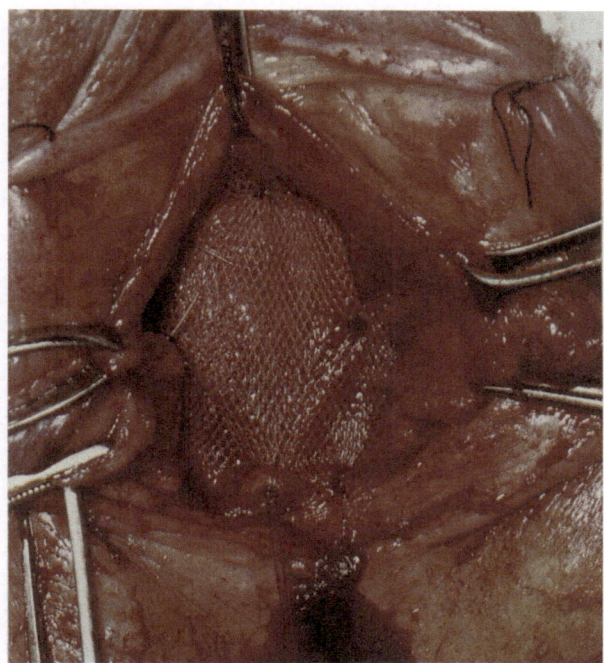

Figure 64. Mersilene mesh reinforcement anchored in position over the re-constituted rectovaginal septum and the reduced enterocoele

such a manner, that the underlying mesh is included with each stitch, continuing to the perineal body.

The perineal body is reconstituted with a No. 1 Vicryl suture on a No. 1 Mayo taper needle which takes a large bite of the levator muscle on one side, passes through the bottom end of the recto-vaginal septal layer, and then the other levator mass. When tied, the levators and rectovaginal septum are pulled together in relation to the external anal sphincter, and the perineal body is reconstituted. The perineal muscles are drawn together with a vertical mattress suture, and finally the vaginal skin closure is completed to the four-chette. A 0.5 cm Penrose drain is inserted into the posterior vaginal wall from the perineal incision, prior to closure with horizontal mattress sutures. A No. 12 Foley catheter is inserted for several days.

This procedure has proved eminently satisfactory with few problems, in a small group of women. One hundred and twenty-two women with a large pulsion enterocoele have been managed since

1968 and of these patients, 25 were treated by total colpocleisis. Early on, some recurrences did occur but with the addition of mersilene mesh no further recurrences have been seen. As the anterior vaginal wall is disturbed very little, longterm urinary symptoms have not been produced. Stress incontinence after colpocleisis of the Neugebauer - Le Fort type doubtless was due to traction in the region of the paraurethral attachment of the posterior pubourethral ligaments — the important part of the suspensory mechanism of the female urethra and the key anatomical site of continence control in the female (Zacharin, 1983). Occasionally stress incontinence is produced following the successful closure of a vesicovaginal fistula, the scarring from this procedure being identical to the distortion produced by post-operative scarring which follows a Neugebauer - Le Fort colpocleisis.

Repair by Combined Abdominal and Vaginal Approach

The great challenge of large pulsion enterocoele to the gynaecological surgeon endeavouring to preserve vaginal function was highlighted by Ridley (1976) in his comments about the three major types of abdominal surgery employed to resuspend and preserve the vagina. The varieties of ventrosuspension, ventrofixation and sacral fixation described numbered 43, yet only relatively few still were mentioned or found a place in current gynaecological surgical texts, indicating that yet another surgical technique was needed to deal with this difficult problem. With the realisation that there were specific anatomical defects present with large pulsion enterocoele, it is remarkable that Ridley's endeavour to tackle the problem with a combined abdomino-vaginal approach is the only paper to advocate this twin-pronged attack since an earlier paper of Zacharin and Hamilton (1972). Ridley's technique used the Masson stripper to take a fascia lata strip which was divided lengthwise. Then the patient was placed in lithotomy position and vaginal hysterectomy performed. Anterior colporrhaphy included a Kelly plication as prophylaxis against stress incontinence, and the enterocoele sac was opened and explored. Immediately prior to obliterating the sac, the fascial strips were sutured firmly to the right and left angles of the vaginal vault, and both long ends passed through the cul-de-sac opening into the peritoneal cavity, then the sac was closed as high as possible. Entering the lower abdomen, the free ends of the straps were identified, led through a tunnel commencing at the internal inguinal ring then fixed without undue tension to the deep surface of the anterior abdominal wall aponeurosis. Finally the Mosch-cowitz procedure was performed.

The result at one year in 12 patients was satisfactory with one recurrent enterocoele not requiring treatment. This composite procedure endeavoured to gain the greatest advantage from three others, namely vaginal repair, ventrosuspension and the Mosch-cowitz. Although a combined abdominovaginal attack, in fact the levator complex wasn't touched and the redundant vagina was sup-ported not over the levator plate to emulate the pelvic cellular tissue effect, but by the anterior abdominal wall. With no further reports on this technique one may assume it has joined the others in relative obscurity.

In 1968, disenchanted with results of available vaginal or abdominal techniques, and cognisant of the work of Berglas and Rubin, an endeavour was made (Zacharin and Hamilton, 1972) to reconstruct or replace the defective anatomy responsible for the appearance of large pulsion enterocoele. This meant levator complex reconstruction with replacement of the upper vagina over a reconstituted levator plate so that rises in intra-abdominal pressure would no longer be able to invert the vagina, through the levator hiatus.

Abdomino-Perineal Repair
of Large Pulsion Enterocoele (A.P.R.E.)

Hughes and Gleadell (1962) reported their experiences in 106 cases of complete rectal prolapse and of these patients, 17 had been managed with a synchronous combined pelvic fascial repair, together with extended perineorrhaphy, and the essential features of their procedure included:

1) dissection and excision of the cul-de-sac,
2) identification of both ureters from the pelvic brim to the broad ligaments, and then clearing the pelvic surface of each levator muscle mass,
3) identification of the levator hiatus from above and below, and its closure by sutures passed from below through the right and left muscle masses, to be tied on the pelvic aspect,
4) obliteration of the denuded pelvic cavity with a series of purse-string sutures, followed by high peritoneal closure and finally,
5) perineorrhaphy.

It seemed this procedure with minor modifications could be ideal to manage large pulsion enterocoele since all the surgical principles required were included and could certainly be effected. The peritoneal sac could be excised completely and both extensive and safe herniorrhaphy performed, which had the effect of retensing the levator crura and plate. With the upper vagina replaced upon the reconstituted plate, to replace pelvic cellular tissue function, minimal vaginal distortion would occur.

The first patient was subjected to this procedure in 1968 and with only minor technical variations, it has continued to the present time. To date 97 women have been treated. Patient reviews were conducted and reported in 1972 and 1979, and more recently a comprehensive follow-up of all patients treated between 1968 and 1984 has been done.

Selection of Patients

Abdominoperineal repair is indicated in patients with a large pulsion enterocoele, who are desirous of retaining normal vaginal function and who enjoy a reasonable state of health. Such patients are in the majority. Unless vaginal function is to be retained, the procedure is not indicated and in elderly females or those in whom general health problems would preclude extensive surgery, colpocleisis has been a most satisfactory alternative. Providing incipient vault ulceration is not present, pre-operative measures should include weight reduction and attention to chronic chest problems especially asthma and chronic bronchitis, so that the best possible clinical state is achieved. It is of especial importance that permanent cessation of cigarette smoking should be promoted actively. Should ulceration be present, vaginal packing is required for two or three days to allow good healing.

Operative Principles

The principles employed in this procedure, based on levator and pelvic cellular tissue defects are as follows:

1) wide excision of the pouch of Douglas;

2) identification of both ureters and the pelvic surface of the levator muscles, then lifting the ureters with their related tissues laterally, well clear of the levator hiatus;

3) identification of both hiatus and crura from above and below;

4) closure of the hiatus by sutures passed through the crura from below, and tied on the pelvic surface;

5) fixing the vaginal vault to the levator plate area, lateral to the rectum;

6) fixing the posterior vaginal wall to the levator closure and reconstituting the introitus.

7) obliteration of the rectovaginal space by a series of purse-string sutures, then peritoneal closure;

Operative Technique

The patient is placed in a lithotomy-Trendelenburg position with the buttocks protruding just over the edge of the operating table. This position permits synchronous access to both abdomen and perineum but although the technique is synchronous, the perineal surgeon should delay his approach in order to minimise blood loss, until the peritoneal sac has been mobilized and the surface of the levator complex identified clearly. The abdominal surgeon enters the peritoneal cavity through a Pfannenstiel or lower paramedian incision and the bowel is packed away. The vaginal vault will be found sagging behind the bladder and prolapsing into the cul-de-sac, its mobility accentuated by the complete absence of the upper normal supports. It is most uncommon to find even a remnant of the lateral pelvic cellular tissues and usually the uterosacral ligaments are of negligible support value also. Should the uterus be present, it is elevated from the operative field and brought forward by guys which attach it to the lower margin of the abdominal

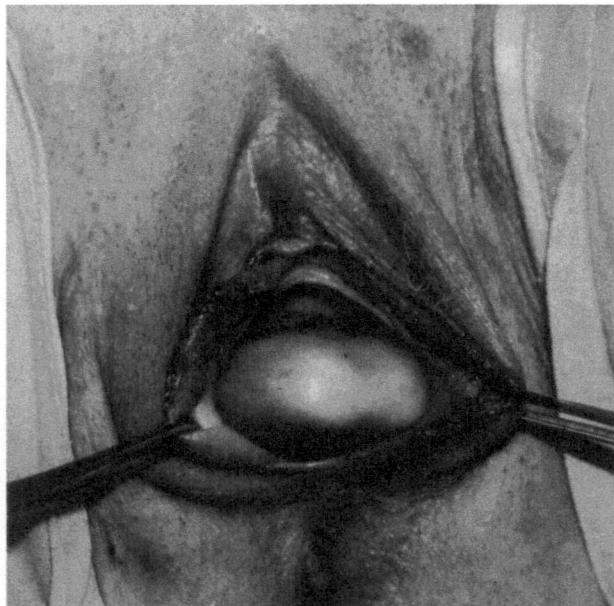

Figure 65 a

Figure 65 a, b. The abdominal surgeon demonstrates the size of the defect

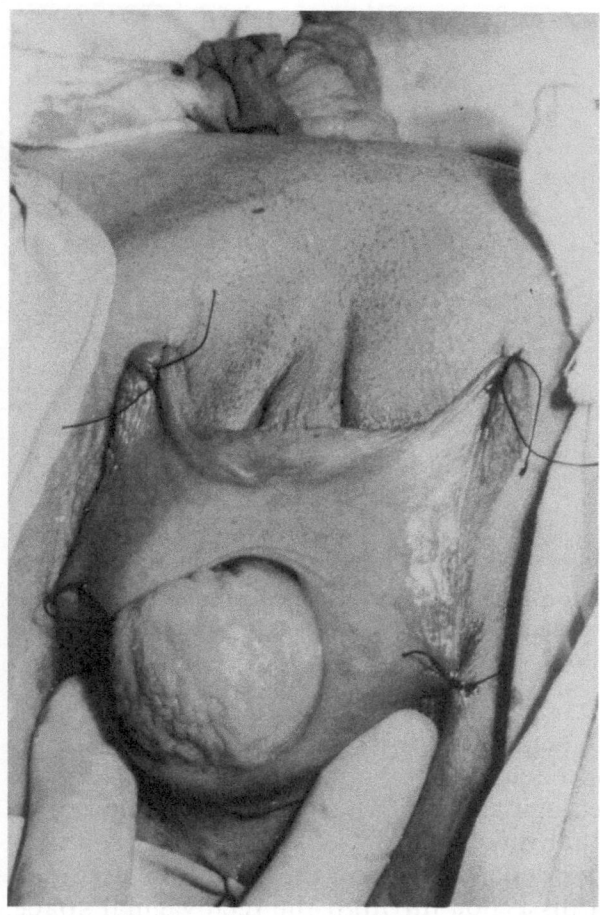

Figure 65 b

wound. When the abdominal surgeon inserts his fingers into the pouch of Douglas, the size of the sac can be demonstrated (Fig. 65 a, b), and he can appreciate the virtual lack of tissues lateral to the neck of the sac.

Both ureters are identified where they cross the pelvic brim, and the peritoneum is divided so they may be traced well forward on the levator muscle. The peritoneal incision begins near the bifurcation of the common iliac artery and extends forward to the cervico-vaginal junction, where it joins the incision from the other side. This forms the lateral and anterior limits for excision of the pouch later in the procedure. When the pouch of Douglas has been mobilized

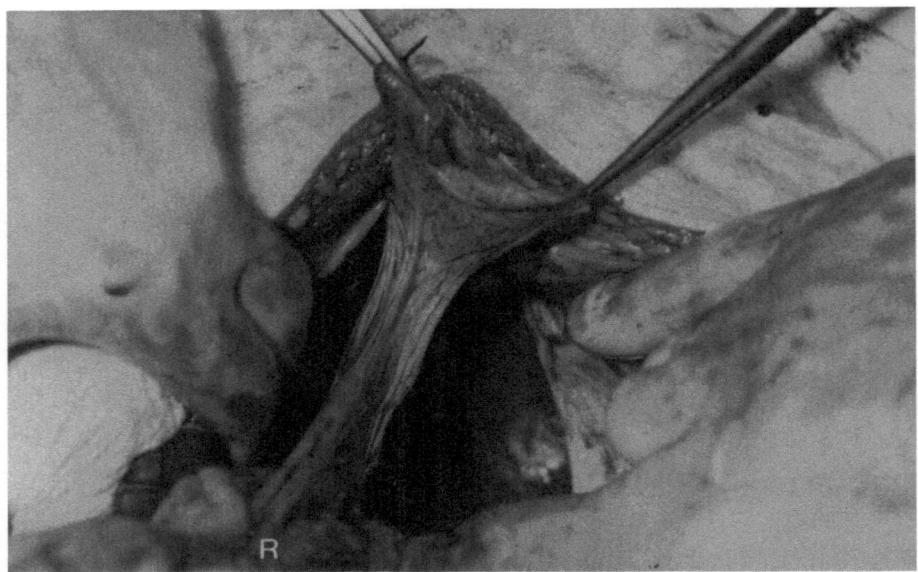

Figure 66. Following wide mobilisation, the peritoneal sac is excised completely by the abdominal surgeon. The rectum *(R)* and the cleared lateral levator areas are demonstrated

and the levators cleared demonstrating both ureters, the perineal surgeon commences approaching the sac along the rectovaginal septum, beginning at the vaginal introitus. The sac is opened, then pulled up by the abdominal surgeon and excised (Fig. 66). A 3 inch wide gauze bandage (1 or 2 depending upon the size of the defect) is passed from the perineal dissection through the rectovaginal space, then tied in front of the pubic symphysis (Fig. 67 a, b). This manoeuvre lifts the bladder and vagina forward against the symphysis, facilitating subsequent final dissection of the levator crura where they attach densely to the anal canal. The angle between the crus and the anal canal accepts the perineal surgeon's index finger, and traction by his finger tenses the muscle.

In every patient the levator ani complex has shown obvious signs of deterioration, most marked in the crural and plate regions. The poor quality muscle may be fibrous, attentuated, splayed and often incomplete. Unilateral absence has been noted on several occasions. So lacking in bulk is the muscle, it is obvious that the likelihood of success in the useful placement of sutures from a vaginal approach

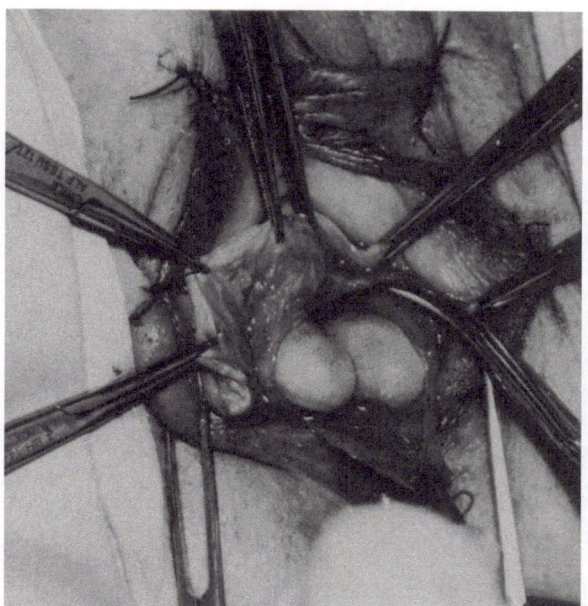

Figure 67 a. Following complete sac excision the adominal surgeon's fingers are seen in the rectovaginal space

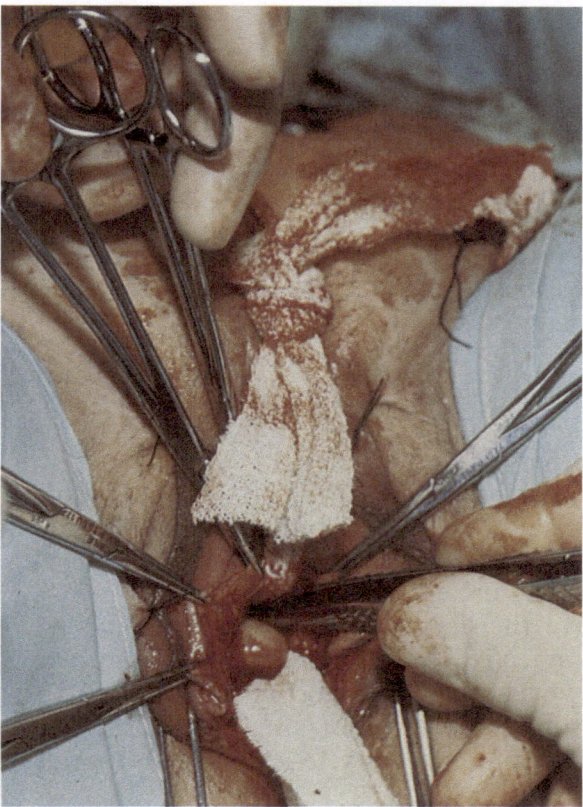

Figure 67 b. The first bandage is in place: the second is placed into the abdominal surgeon's fingers

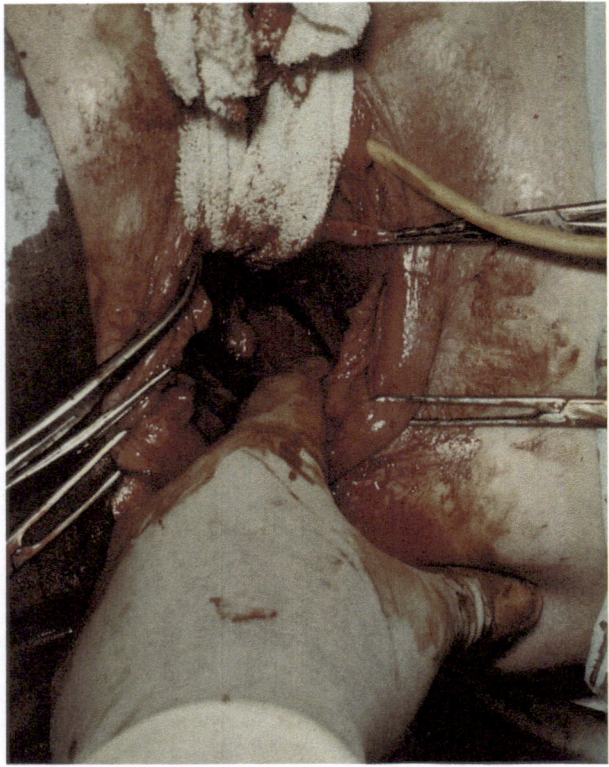

Figure 68. The perineal surgeon tenses the levator crus by exerting traction with his index finger hooked into the angle between the rectum and the levator

alone would be minimal, and a great advantage of the combined approach can be appreciated. Additionally, a common finding after previous vaginal hysterectomy is the much more medial position adopted by one or both ureters, rendering them at some risk from a blind vaginal placement of sutures. The combined approach enables large safe bites of levator tissue to be taken and approximated, with the certain knowledge that the ureters are safe.

It is important to move the ureters out of the operative field along with their related connective tissue, which contains important nerve supply from the hypogastric plexus destined for the bladder. This manoeuvre may help minimize the entrapment of these nerve fibres in the levator crural closure, thereby lessening post-operative

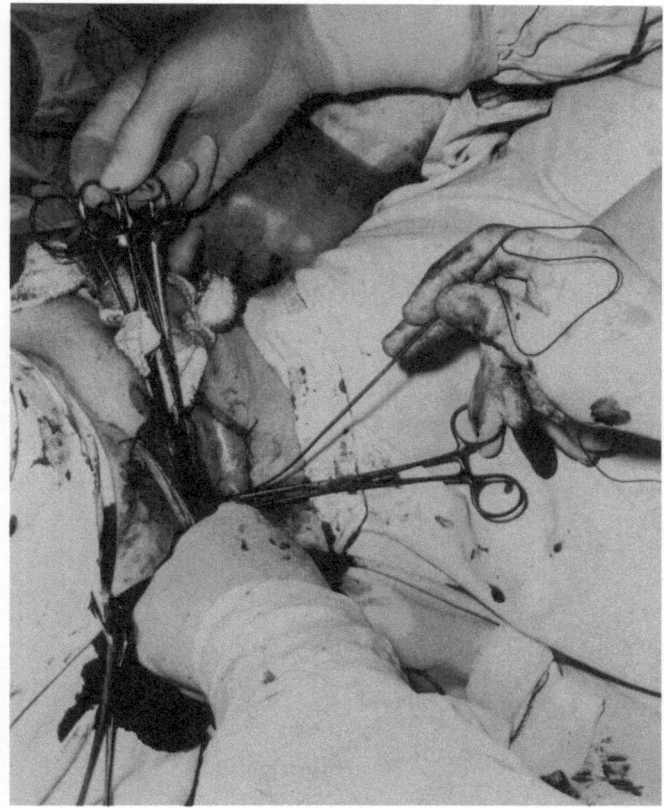

Figure 69 a

Figure 69 a, b. The passage of the long needle on the patient's left side **(a)**. The index finger tenses the levator to aid needle placement and also protects the anal canal from any possible damage. The close up **(b)** shows greater detail including the passage of the needle through the vaginal skin

urinary retention, and bladder problems have been less troublesome since the ureter has been transposed en masse with its surrounding connective tissues. If the ureter is well clear of the operative field when first exposed, no transposition is necessary. With the ureters clear of the operative field, the perineal surgeon tenses the crus by traction in the angle between the muscle and anal canal (Fig. 68). A long needle with a slight terminal curve carrying a no 2 chromic catgut suture is passed through vaginal skin, describes an arc toward the lateral pelvic wall to pick up as much levator tissue as is safe, but always under the watchful eye and verbal guidance of the

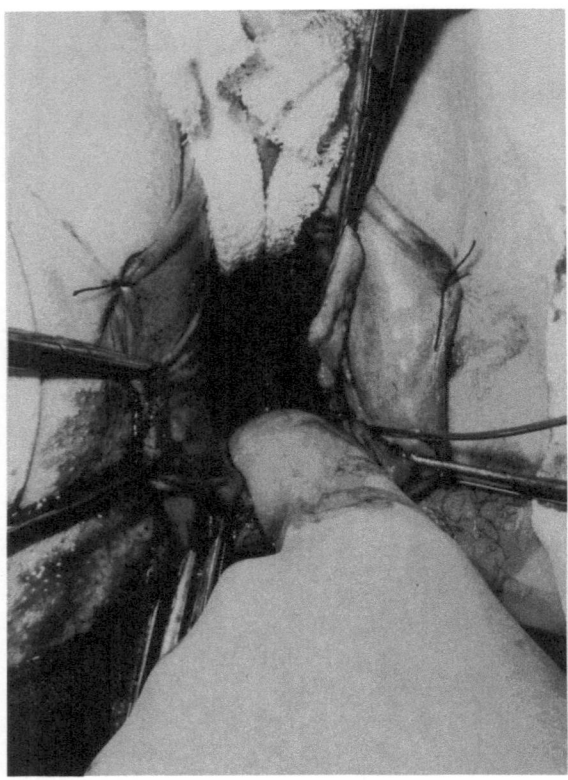

Figure 69 b

abdominal surgeon. In this way the surgeon can pick up a very large
block of muscle tissue, knowing the ureter is clear (Fig. 69 a, b, c, d).

The needle is grasped by the abdominal surgeon when its point is
seen and its passage through the muscle is completed. The catgut is
drawn after it and the abdominal surgeon unthreads the needle, to
return it to the perineal surgeon, who reloads the other end of the
suture to complete the stitch by passing the needle through vaginal
epithelium and levator muscle of the opposite side (Fig. 70). Usually
3 such sutures are necessary, occasionally 4 depending upon the size
of the defect. Elevating the sutures by the abdominal surgeon,
enables him to decide how many more would be required (Fig. 71 a,
b, c). Closure should not constrict either rectum or vagina. Now the
bandage is cut and removed, and the perineal surgeon pushes up the
apex of the vaginal vault so the abdominal surgeon may grasp it, for
it is important that the tip of the vault is identified accurately, ready

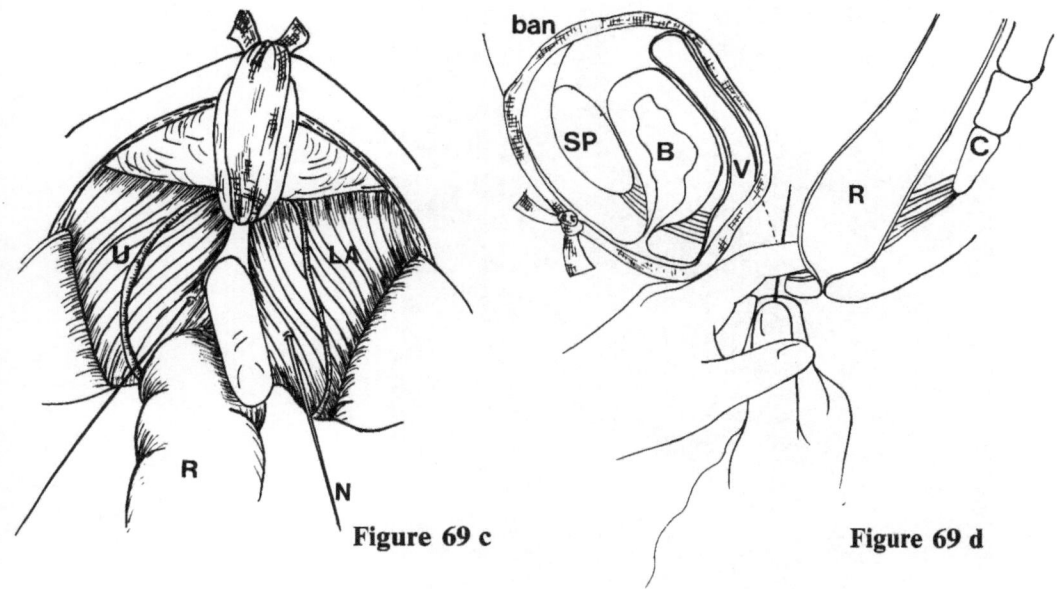

Figure 69 c

Figure 69 d

Figure 69 c, d. Two line drawings of the situation in Figure 69 a, b.
c is the view from above showing the index finger between the levator
crura, pushing aside the anal canal and tensing the crus. Passage of the
suture on the left side has been completed and the needle is seen coming
through the right levator crus. Both ureters are well clear.
d is a sagittal view showing bladder and vagina drawn forward by the
bandage, the finger tensing the crus and the needle passing through the
right levator crus.
V vagina; R rectum; SP symphysis pubis; U ureter; ban bandage; LA
levator ani; N needle; C coccyx; B bladder

for future placement on the reconstituted levator plate. Now the
epithelium of the posterior vaginal wall is closed using no 0 Dexon
on a no 3 curved Mayo trocar needle. A running locking suture is
chosen, the surgeon being careful that each skin bite includes underlying levator tissues and fascia to ensure close adhesion of the
vaginal wall to levator tissue, which is reinforced further when the
crural sutures are tied later. Rarely is it necessary to excise
redundant vaginal epithelium, for experience has shown that the
redundancy disappears with time. The perineal body is reconstituted, a long 1 cm Penrose rubber drain is passed into the rectovaginal space and the perineal skin closed. A no 12 Foley/self-

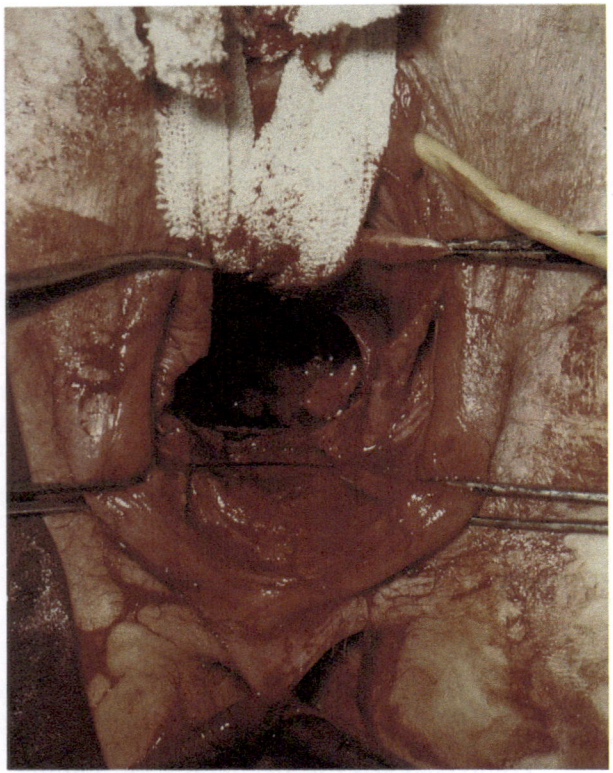

Figure 70. The first completed suture. Note the large blocks of tissue, vaginal epithelium and levator, picked up on either side

retaining catheter is inserted and rectal examination performed to exclude damage.

After the vaginal epithelium has been reconstituted, the abdominal surgeon ties the sutures to approximate the levator crura, for should this be done earlier, the perineal surgeon would experience great difficulty closing the vaginal epithelium, such is the elevation produced when the crura are united. Following crural closure, the intercrural space immediately anterior to the rectum is inspected. Should there be any inadequacy in approximation of the crura, several sutures of no 2 chromic catgut are inserted to complete crural closure and eliminate any space in front of the rectum. Crural closure should fit snugly against the rectal wall but not exert a constricting effect (Fig. 72).

After the completion of crural closure, the vaginal vault is fixed

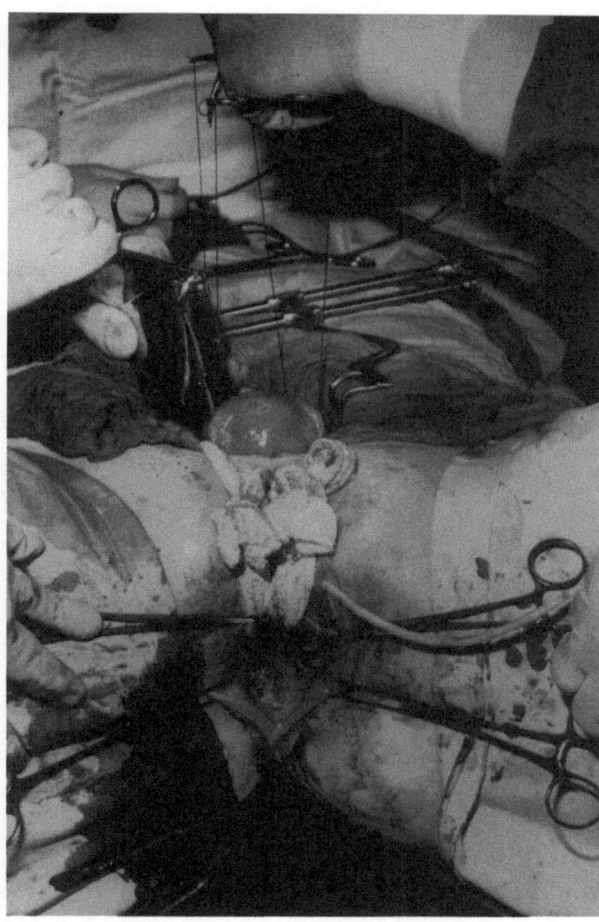

Figure 71 a. The abdominal surgeon elevates the levator sutures in order to assess the adequacy of crural apposition

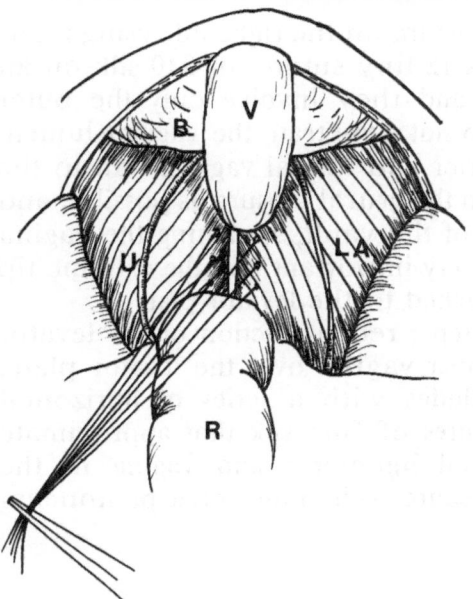

Figure 71 b. Diagrammatic representation of **Figure 71 a**: *V* vagina; *R* rectum; *LA* levator ani; *U* ureter; *B* bladder

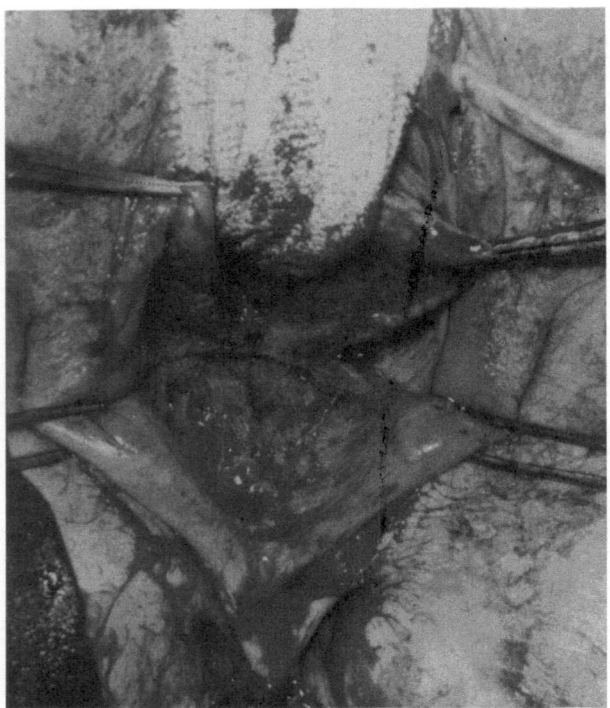

Figure 71 c. The levator masses with overlying vaginal epithelium are drawn together by elevation of the sutures

to the levator plate lateral to the rectum on the right side using interrupted sutures. Often as many as 12 tiny sutures of 3/0 silk on an atraumatic needle are required and they involve only the outer layers of the vaginal wall and do not penetrate the vaginal lumen. The sutures pass from the posterior and lateral vaginal wall to the plate muscle, beginning as near to the crural closure as possible and gradually advance up to the tip of the vault, stretching the vagina onto the plate (Fig. 73 a, b). It is very important that the extreme tip of the vault should be firmly attached to the levator plate.

These then are the two key steps: reconstruction of the levator defect, and placement of the upper vagina over the levator plate. The abdominal procedure concludes with a series of horizontal obliterating 3/0 purse-string sutures of fine silk that approximate the lower rectal wall, uterosacral ligaments and vagina in the manner of the Moschcowitz procedure. When the pelvic peritoneum

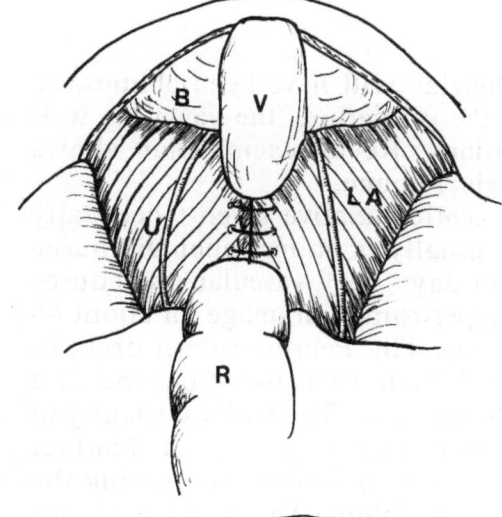

Figure 72. Diagram of completed crural closure.
R rectum; *U* ureter; *V* vagina; *B* bladder; *LA* levator ani

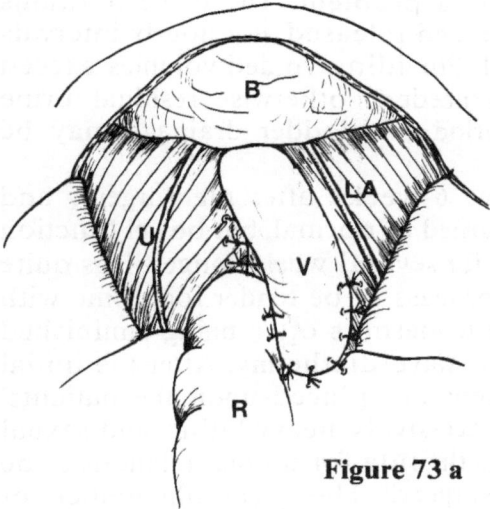

Figure 73 a, b. Line drawings showing the upper vagina including the extreme tip, fixed to the crus and plate by a series of fine silk sutures.
a View from above. **b** The lateral view.
B bladder; *V* vagina; *SP* symphysis pubis; *U* ureter; *R* rectum; *LA* levator ani; *C* coccyx

Figure 73 a

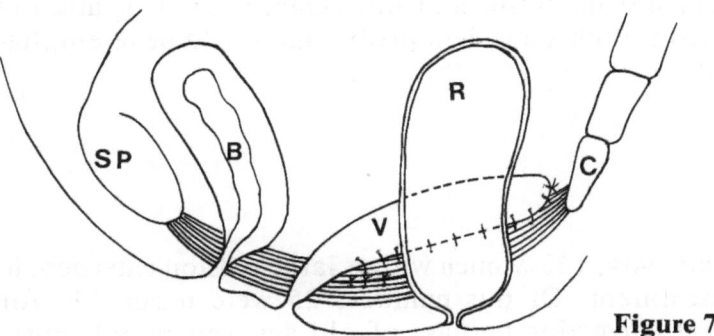

Figure 73 b

has been closed, the pouch of Douglas will have been obliterated completely. At the conclusion of the procedure, the vagina is well supported and of normal dimensions. Rectal examination shows firm tissue support in the rectovaginal space.

Bowel function assisted by a gentle laxative given twice daily from the third post-operative day, usually is normal upon discharge from hospital on the 12th or 14th day. Very vascular procedures have required vacuum suction retroperitoneal drainage for about 48 hours but this is necessary only rarely. The Penrose rubber drain in the rectovaginal space is shortened 2 cm each day from the 2nd post-operative day until it is finally removed. The major difficulty in the post-operative period has been the regaining of bladder function, but since more care has been exercised in transposing the ureters, this has been much less a problem. The catheter drains freely for 3 days then is clamped and released at 4 hourly intervals for 24 hours prior to its removal. Providing voided volumes exceed 200 ml, no further attention is needed, otherwise residual urine determinations or a further period of bladder drainage may be necessary.

Post-operative review is done 6 weeks after the surgery, and usually bladder function has returned to normal, but bowel function may still require a mild laxative for several weeks longer. It is quite usual for the reconstituted levator mass to be tender for a time with gradual improvement, persistent tenderness often being diminished greatly by the use of pelvic short wave diathermy. After the initial post-operative visit, no restrictions are placed upon the patients' activities with the exception of excessively heavy lifting, and sexual intercourse may be resumed. It is the rule for normal relations to be occurring 8—10 weeks from surgery. The great importance of long-term weight control, abstinence from cigarette smoking and the careful management of chronic chest problems should be re-emphasized at this visit.

Results

Between 1968 and 1984, 122 women with a large pulsion enterocoele presented for treatment. Of this number, 25 were unsuitable for abdominoperineal correction because of old age, general infirmity, or the fact that sexual intercourse was no longer required. This group of 25 women were managed by colpocleisis with excellent long-term benefits and minimal operative or convalescent problems. As already indicated, there were several recurrences early in the series, but following the addition of a mersilene mesh insert, there have been no further problems. Ninety-seven women have undergone abdominoperineal repair during the last 17 years, and accurate follow-up of this group was completed on the 30th June, 1984. Difficulties with follow-up have been due to the time interval since 1968 and also the fact that some patients have come great distances, from every state in Australia. Previous surveys of this procedure were published in 1972 and 1980, and the long-term benefits evident from this present follow-up indicates that a similar trend to those earlier reports has been maintained (Table I).

Table I

Year	No. of Pat.	No. of Previous Operations						Recurrent Enterocoele	Recurrent Cystocoele	Lost to Follow-up	Cure	Fail
		0	1	2	3	4	5					
1968	2		2								2	
1969	2		1	1						1	1	
1970	3		2	1						1	2	
1971	10		5	4	1					5	5	
1972	2		2							1	1	
1973	4		3		1				2		4	
1974	4		1	3						1	3	
1975	10		8	2				2	2	2	6	2
1976	9		4	4	1			3		1	5	3
1977	6		5	1						2	4	
1978	6		5	1						1	5	
1979	15	1	9	4	1			1	3	3	12	1
1980	6	1	3	1	1				1	1	5	
1981	5		2	3				1			4	1
1982	5		3	2						1	4	
1983	4		2		2						4	
1984	4		1	1	2						4	
Total	97	2	55	29	10		1	7	8	20	70	7

97

Of 97 patients managed by abdominoperineal repair, 20 could not be traced leaving 77 to be reviewed. During the period 1968—1984, 70 women have been cured, the more recent patients for a short time only but experience has shown clearly that should recurrence occur it does so quickly after the surgery. Most of these women had suffered recurrent enterocoele after former attempts at correction, so in fact they have acted as their own controls — providing they stay cured for six months, the result appears to be permanent. It should be appreciated that the 9 patients lost to follow-up in this present review from the years 1969—1979 were in fact listed as cures in the 1980 review.

Cure means an absence of any pulsion enterocoele, a normally supported vagina and normal sexual intercourse. There have been 7 known enterocoele recurrences, 6 occurred relatively early in the series and one more recently in 1981. All 97 patients showed poor quality pelvic tissues at surgery and the worse the tissues the more difficult it was to effect levator hiatal closure and restoration of levator plate function, yet in a majority, enough tissue could be drawn across the midline to close the hiatus effectively and produce some sort of levator plate. No doubt the ability to recreate this failed anatomy increased with surgical experience.

In every instance of recurrence, the problem has been identical — the vaginal vault has drawn away from the poor levator plate tissues, so it can no longer be supported effectively during rises in intra-abdominal pressure, and therefore vaginal inversion recommences. The speed of recurrence and development of the enterocoele seems directly related to operative problems encountered in patients with extremely poor tissues, and difficulties in producing an adequate levator plate. All the recurrences have been corrected by abdominal intervention alone, reinforcing the plate area with mersilene mesh and repositioning the vaginal vault into its correct situation over the plate. The 1979 recurrence is tiny and associated with a large rectocoele which occurred during a recent episode of prolonged constipation.

Recurrent cystocoele really is a misnomer, because surgery is usually not performed upon the anterior vaginal wall during enterocoele repair, since as explained already, in most instances the lax vaginal epithelium "takes up" after enterocoele correction, and the anterior vaginal wall bulge disappears. Since urinary symptoms are uncommon in the primary presentation, it is likely that any anterior vaginal wall bulge is secondary to the vault inversion, and not really a true cystocoele. Also it is difficult to decide just how much redundant and stretched anterior vaginal wall epithelium should be removed, for over-enthusiastic removal can produce stenosis in association with the completion of post-operative involution. The anterior vaginal wall is corrected at primary surgery only when there is gross laxity, or if gravitationally induced bladder symptoms were present before, otherwise a "wait and see" approach seems best.

There have been 8 cystocoeles detected since enterocoele correction, yet only 4 have required further surgery because of symptoms and the others are being reviewed at regular intervals.

The accompanying table of results shows that every patient, with the exception of two, had preceding pelvic surgery and in 40 women more than one previous pelvic operation. Vaginal hysterectomy was the primary procedure in 45 patients, Manchester repair in 31 and

Table II
Type of Primary Pelvic Surgery

Year	Vaginal Hysterectomy	Abdominal Hysterectomy	Manchester
1968			2
1969			2
1970		1	2
1971	2		8
1972	2		
1973	3		1
1974	1	2	1
1975	4	4	2
1976	6	3	
1977	2	1	3
1978	5	1	
1979	8	1	5
1980	4	1	
1981	1	2	2
1982	2	1	2
1983	2	1	1
1984	3	1	
Total	45	19	31

95

abdominal hysterectomy in 19 (Table II). The most common second and third procedures were repeat vaginal repairs of various types. The two patients without previous pelvic surgery were a young women of 25 years and an elderly woman of 63 years. The young woman, seen in 1979, had been involved in a motor-bike accident 2 years previously during her first pregnancy, at 14 weeks gestation. The pelvis, right femur and left forearm were fractured together with a very deep laceration involving the right greater labium and extending deeply into the right lateral vaginal wall. There was associated wide separation of the pubic symphysis. The deep laceration was explored and closed with drainage but because of the pregnancy the femur was treated with traction and the pelvis supported in a sling. She did not become ambulant until 36 weeks gestation

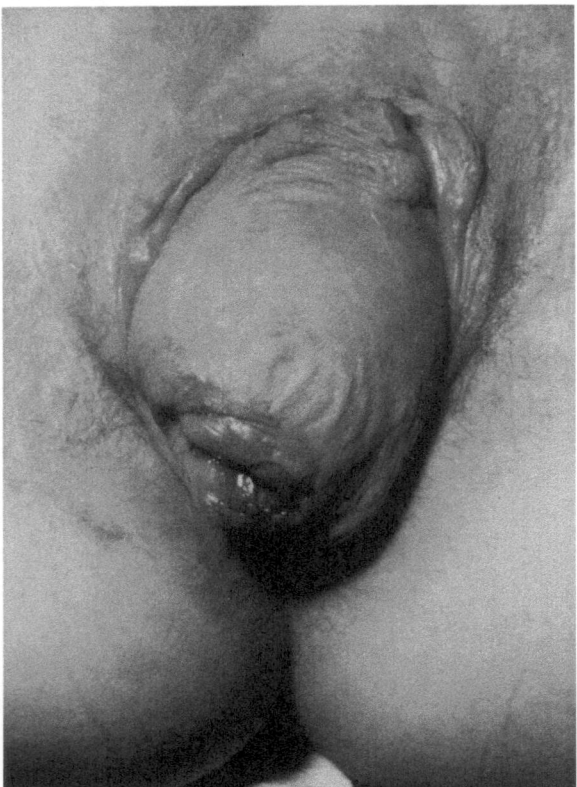

Figure 74. The procidentia which developed following pelvic trauma. The large enterocoele sac can be seen behind the cervix

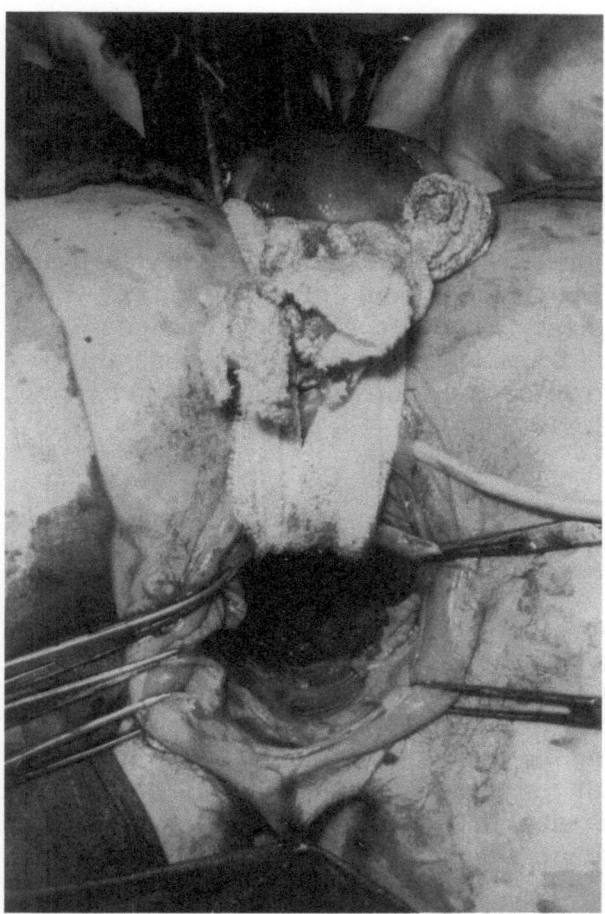

Figure 75. The large pelvic floor defect following pelvic disruption and levator ani damage

when a marked genital prolapse was noted for the first time. The cervix protruded through the introitus, the foetal head could be palpated with ease and a comment was made that no muscular resistance was present in the anterior and posterior pelvis. The subsequent vaginal delivery was uneventful but later an attempt to mobilise the right sacroiliac joint failed so the symphyseal diastasis of about 9 cm persisted. The prolapse worsened in degree and examination demonstrated a procidentia with an evident large enterocoele sac (Fig. 74). It was surmised that both the deep vaginal laceration and damage to her bony pelvis had torn and disrupted the levator mechanism on the injured side, the situation being accentuated by the effect of the pregnancy.

At abdominoperineal repair the levator of that side was almost absent and replaced by poor quality scar tissue. A huge pelvic floor defect was evident when the bandages were put in place (Fig. 75) and with some difficulty the levator hiatus was closed, producing a fair levator plate. The plate was reinforced by mersilene mesh and the vault secured to it. The result has remained good but has yet to withstand a second pregnancy. The elderly female presented in 1980 with a huge procidentia. Correction was attempted by abdominoperineal attack in association with and following a Manchester repair. The result has remained good.

Complications

In this series of 97 women there have been three serious complications, all early in the series, suggesting that increased experience minimises the risk of such problems. The rectum was perforated on two occasions, once by each operator but the defects were recognized and closed allowing the procedure to be completed and rectal healing occurred without further incident. It is usual for the anal canal to be densely adherent to the lower posterior vaginal wall after many vaginal repairs and great care must be taken during dissection. Sharp dissection with scissors is the safest way to proceed, the vaginal epithelium being stretched over the fingers of one hand, enabling the junction of anal canal and epithelium to be detected more readily, prior to their separation. The rectum commonly is thin walled and densely adherent to surrounding structures in these women especially after multiple attempts at correction and the abdominal surgeon must proceed with great care, drawing the rectum up and putting it on the stretch, to facilitate its mobilisation. The situation is improved greatly following placement of the bandages which draw the vagina and bladder forward, and the perineal surgeon can help his colleague by tensing the levator crus first on one side then the other, with the index finger in the angle between the rectum and the levator. The rectum must be mobilised down to the levator hiatus.

In 1971, on the.8th post-operative day, a sudden rectal haemorrhage occurred which subsided spontaneously but required transfusion. Later investigation was unrewarding and showed some mild congestion of the rectal mucosa. There have been no similar incidents since then and perhaps its cause might have been a badly placed levator suture. It is important to perform rectal examination after hiatal closure to be sure the rectum is undamaged.

All procedures reported, which attempt correction of large pulsion enterocoele, have produced their share of complications, many serious and so it seems the small number that have occurred in this series is acceptable when dealing with such a formidable problem. As the figures indicate, experience with the procedure and care in pelvic dissection may reduce important complications to zero.

Conclusions

Large pulsion enterocoele is a difficult surgical problem. If correction is to provide adequate duration of cure and restore normal vaginal function, the technique chosen must be based upon sound anatomical facts. Most available procedures fail in both respects. Pulsion enterocoele occurs because of a combination of changes in both the pelvic cellular tissues and the levator ani muscle complex. The synchronous abdominoperineal technique attends to both defects. For the patient able to tolerate major surgery and desirous of regaining normal vaginal function, this combined approach offers many anatomical and therapeutic advantages. A majority of women with the problem fall into this category and the others are managed best by local vaginal surgery or total colpocleisis. In a series of 97 patients treated in the past 17 years, careful follow-up has been possible in 77 and 70 are known to be cured. It should be remembered that a high proportion of these patients had experienced repeated failures from other techniques. The abdominoperineal approach to large pulsion enterocoele is a safe procedure and with experience, virtually free from serious complications. It offers a very high long-term cure rate together with restoration of normal vaginal function.

Bibliography

Ajabor, L. N., Okojie, S. E.: Genital prolapse in the newborn. Int. Surg. *61*, 496—497 (1976).

Al-Rawi, Z. S., Al-Rawi, Z. T.: Joint hypermobility in women with genital prolapse. Lancet *1*, 1439—1441 (1982).

Amico, J. C., Marino, A. W.: Prolapse of the vagina in association with rectal procidentia. Dis. Colon Rectum *11*, 115—119 (1968).

Amreich, J.: Aetiologie und Operation des Scheidenstumpfprolapses. Wien. klin. Wschr. *63*, 74—77 (1951).

Anderson, W. R.: Pudendal hernia: Unusual cause of labial mass. Obstet. Gynec. *32*, 802—804 (1968).

Ardekany, M. S., Rafee, R.: A new modification of colpocleisis for treatment of total procidentia in old age. Int. J. Gynaec. Obstet. *15*, 358—360 (1978).

Arthure, H. G. E., Savage, D.: Uterine prolapse and prolapse of the vaginal vault treated by sacral hysteropexy. Br. J. Obstet. Gynaec. *69*, 355—360 (1957).

Austin, R. C., Damstra, E. F.: New fascia plastic repair of enterocoele. Surg. Gynec. Obstet. *104*, 297—304 (1957).

Ayoub, S. F.: The anterior fibres of the levator ani muscle in man. J. Anat. *128*, 571—580 (1979).

Azpuru, C. E.: Total rectal prolapse and total genital prolapse. Dis. Colon Rectum *17*, 528—531 (1974).

Barker, F.: Vaginal hernia or enterocoele. Am. J. Obstet. Surg. *9*, 177—192 (1876).

Barrett, C. W.: Hernias through the pelvic floor. Amer. J. Obstet. Gynec. *59*, 553—569 (1909).

Beecham, C. T., Beecham, J. B.: Correction of prolapsed vagina or enterocoele with fascia lata. Obstet. Gynec. *42*, 542—546 (1973).

Berg, R. A.: Labial hernia: demonstration by herniography. A. J. R. *133*, 138—139 (1979).

Berglas, B., Rubin, I. C.: Histologic study of the pelvic connective tissue Surg. Gynec. Obstet. *97*, 277—289 (1953).

Berglas, B., Rubin, I. C.: Study of the supportive structures of the uterus by levator myography. Surg. Gynec. Obstet. *97*, 677—692 (1953).

Berkeley, C., Bonney, V.: Gynecological surgery. New York: Paul Hoeber Inc. 1948.

Birchenall, J.: Vaginal hernia; perforation of ileum under sudden violence. Br. Med. J. 2, 182—183 (1869).

Birnbaum, S. J.: Rational therapy for the prolapsed vagina. Amer. J. Obstet. Gynec. 115, 411—419 (1973).

Brady, L.: An operation to correct genital prolapse following vaginal pan-hysterectomy. Amer. J. Obstet. Gynec. 32, 295—299 (1936).

Bremer, E. H.: Prolapse of the vagina following total hysterectomy. Arch. Surg. 92, 20—22 (1966).

Bueermann, W. H.: Vaginal enterocoele: report of three cases. JAMA 99, 1138—1143 (1932).

Burch, J. C.: Urethrovaginal fixation to Cooper's ligament for correction of stress incontinence, cystocoele and prolapse. Amer. J. Obstet. Gynec. 81, 281—290 (1961).

Campbell, R. M.: The anatomy and histology of the sacrouterine ligaments. Amer. J. Obstet. Gynec. 59, 1—12 (1950).

Chan, P. L., Neale, R.: Spontaneous rupture of the vaginal vault with small bowel prolapse. Obstet. Gynec. 60, 754 (1982).

Chase, H. C.: Levator hernia (pudendal hernia). Surg. Gynec. Obstet. 35, 717—732 (1922).

Cottom, D., Williams, E.: Procidentia in the newborn. Br. J. Obstet. Gynaec. 72, 131—136 (1965).

Cowan, W., Morgan, H. R.: Abdominal sacral colpopexy. Amer. J. Obstet. Gynec. 138, 348—350 (1980).

Cox, P. S. V., Webster, D.: Genital prolapse amongst the Pokot. E. Afr. med. J. 52, 694—699 (1975).

Critchley, H. O. D., Dixon, J. S., Gosling, J. A.: Comparative study of the periurethral and perianal parts of the human levator ani muscle. Urol. Int. 35, 226—232 (1980).

Cuneo, B., Veau, V.: De la signification morphologique des aponeuroses périvésicales. J. Anat. 35, 235—245 (1899).

Curtis, A. H., Anson, B. J., Beaton, L. E.: The anatomy of the subperitoneal tissues and ligamentous structures in relation to surgery of the female pelvic viscera. Surg. Gynec. Obstet. 70, 643—656 (1940).

Dastur, B., Gurubaxani, G., Palnitkar, S. S.: Shirodkar sling operation in the treatment of genital prolapse. J. Obstet. Gynaec. Brit. Emp. 74, 125—128 (1967).

Davies, J. W.: Man's assumption of the erect posture — Its effect on the position of the pelvis. Amer. J. Obstet. Gynec. 70, 1012—1020 (1955).

Derry, D. E.: On the real nature of the so-called "pelvic fascia". J. Anat. Physiol. 42, 97—106 (1907—1908).

Derry, D. E.: Pelvic muscles and fasciae. J. Anat. Physiol. *42*, 107—111 (1907—1908).

Dickinson, R. L.: The vagina as a hernial canal. Amer. J. Obstet. Dis. Wom. & Child. *22*, 692—697 (1889).

Diddle, A. W.: Partial colpocleisis for complete vaginal prolapse: demonstration of a technic. J. Reprod. Med. *4*, 33—35 (1970).

Elftman, H. O.: The evolution of the pelvic floor of primates. Am. J. Anat. *51*, 307—346 (1932).

El-Kholi, G. Y., Mina, S. N.: Elastic tissue of the vagina in genital prolapse. J. Egypt. med. Ass. *58*, 196—204 (1975).

Embrey, M. P.: An abdominal sling operation for the repair of enterocoele and vault prolapse. J. Obstet. Gynaec. Brit. Emp. *68*, 471—474 (1961).

Emge, L. A., Durfee, R. B.: Pelvic organ prolapse: four thousand years of treatment. Clin. Obstet. Gynec. *9*, 997—1032 (1966).

Falk, H. C.: Uterine prolapse and prolapse of the vaginal vault treated by sacroperxy. Obstet. Gynec. *18*, 113—115 (1961).

Falk, H. C., Kaufman, S.: Partial colpocleisis: The Le Fort procedure (analysis of 100 cases). Obstet. Gynec. *5*, 617—627 (1955).

Fanciulli, S., Ragaglini, G., Ternelli, F.: Un caso di enterocele vaginale. Minerva Ginec. *27*, 1060—1067 (1975).

Feldman, G. B., Birnbaum, S. J.: Sacral colpopexy for vaginal vault prolapse. Obstet. Gynec. *53*, 399—401 (1979).

Ferguson, W. H.: New functional repair of post-hysterectomy vaginal vault prolapse with Marlex Mesh. Amer. Surg. *30*, 227—230 (1964).

Feroze, R. M.: Vaginal hysterectomy and repair. Clin. Obstet. Gynaec. *5*, 545—556 (1978).

Findley, P.: Prolapse of the uterus in nulliparous women. Amer. J. Obstet. Dis. Wom. *75*, 12—21 (1917).

Fiske-Jones, D.: Relation of the deep cul-de-sac to prolapse of the rectum and uterus, and to rectocele. Boston Med. Surg. J. *175*, 623—627 (1916).

Fletcher, P. F.: Abdominal colpocystopexy for complete prolapse of the vagina and bladder: the rectus suspension principle of crossed-suspender support. Amer. J. Obstet. Gynec. *56*, 41—59 (1948).

Fothergill, W. E.: The supports of the pelvic viscera: a review of some recent contributions to pelvic anatomy, with a clinical introduction. J. Obstet. Gynaec. Brit. Emp. *13*, 18—28 (1908).

Fraenkel, L.: The principles of the treatment of genital prolapse: the technic of ventrofixation of the vagina. Amer. J. Obstet. Gynec. *13*, 757—759 (1927).

Frank, R. T.: A study of the anatomy pathology and treatment of uterine prolapse, rectocele and cystocele. Surg. Gynec. Obstet. *24*, 42—60 (1917).

Friedman, E. A., Meltzer, R. M.: Collagen mesh prosthesis for repair of endopelvic fascial defects. Amer. J. Obstet. Gynec. *106*, 430—433 (1970).

Gallo, D.: Commentary on the work — "Use of Cooper's ligament and the mersilene band". Ginecol. Obstet. Mex. *21*, 957—961 (1966).

Geary, W. L.: The superior vaginal segment — uterine prolapse. Clin. Obstet. Gynaec. *15*, 1133—1144 (1972).

Goff, B. H.: A practical consideration of the damaged pelvic floor with a technique for its secondary reconstruction. Surg. Gynec. Obstet. *46*, 855—866 (1928).

Goff, B. H.: An histological study of the perivaginal fascia in a nullipara. Surg. Gynec. Obstet. *52*, 32—42 (1931).

Goldman, J., Ovadia, J., Feldberg, D.: The Neugebauer - Le Fort Operation: A review of 118 partial colpocleises. Eur. J. Obstet. Gynec. Reprod. Biol. *12*, 31—35 (1981).

Goodall, J. R., Power, R. M. H.: A modification of the Le Fort operation for increasing its scope. Amer. J. Obstet. Gynec. *34*, 968—976 (1937).

Graham, W., Clegg, J. F., Taylor, V.: Complete rectal prolapse: repair by a simple technique. Ann. R. Coll. Surg. Engl. *66*, 87—89 (1984).

Grunberger, V.: Promontoriofixur bei Prolaps des Scheidenblindsackes. Wien. klin. Wschr. *88*, 324—325 (1976).

Guiou, N. M.: Fascial suspension of the vagina. Can. J. Surg. *60*, 600—602 (1949).

Halban, J., Tandler, J.: Anatomie und Aetiologie der Genital-Prolapse beim Weibe. Wien: W. Braumüller 1907.

Hanson, G. E. Keettel, W. C.: The Neugebauer - Le Fort operation: a review of 288 colpocleises. Obstet. Gynec. *34*, 352—357 (1969).

Hawksworth, W., Roux, J. P.: Vaginal hysterectomy. J. Obstet. Gynaec. Brit. Emp. *65*, 214—218 (1958).

Heaney, N. S.: Vaginal hysterectomy in cure of prolapsus uteri. Amer. J. Surg. *33*, 471—473 (1936).

Herman, G.: Pudendal (Labial) hernia. N. Engl. J. Med. *265*, 435—436 (1961).

Hill, E. C., Hoag, R. W.: Experience with the Manchester operation. Surg. Gynec. Obstet. *104*, 167—175 (1957).

Hiller, R. I.: Repair of enterocele with preservation of the vagina. Amer. J. Obstet. Gynec. *64*, 409—412 (1952).

Holl, K. B. von: Handbuch der Anatomie des Menschen. Jena: Fischer 1897.

Holland, J. B.: Enterocele and prolapse of the vaginal vault. Clin. Obstet. Gynec. *15*, 1145—1154 (1972).

Hughes, E. S R., Gleadell, L. W.: Prolapse of the rectum. Proc. R. Soc. Med. *55*, 1077—1080 (1962).

Inmon, W. B.: Suspension of the vaginal cuff and posterior repair following vaginal hysterectomy. Amer. J. Obstet. Gynec. *120*, 977—982 (1974).

Inmon, W. B., Bledsoe, J. W.: Surgical repair of genital prolapse after hemipelvectomy. Amer. J. Obstet. Gynec. *123*, 766—769 (1975).

Jarcho, J.: Vaginopexy or ventrofixation of the vagina: A simple operation for the cure of prolapse of the uterus and cystocoele. Clin. Med. & Surg. *35*, 555—558 (1928).

Jeannel, D.: Du prolapsus du rectum. Clin. Fact. Med. Toulouse 1896, *11*, 101—121 (1896).

Jones, D. F.: Relation of the deep cul-de-sac to prolapse of the rectum and uterus, and to rectocoele. Boston Med. Surg. J. *175*, 623—627 (1916).

Jones, H. W., jr.: Editorial comment. Obstet. Gynec. Surv. *29*, 93 (1974).

Jones, H. W., jr.: Editorial comment. Obstet. Gynec. Surv. *37*, 351 (1982).

Kaskarelis, D. B.: An abdominal approach to the surgical repair of post-hysterectomy vaginal inversion. Acta Obstet. Gynec. Scand. *57*, 173—175 (1978).

Keith, A.: Human Embryology and Morphology. London: Arnold 1902.

Kinzel, G. E.: Enterocele: A study of 265 cases. Amer. J. Obstet. Gynec. *81*, 1166—1174 (1961).

Kocks, J.: Die normale und physiologische Lage und Gestalt des Uterus sowie deren Mechanik. Bonn: Max Cohen & Sohn 1880.

Koontz, A. R.: Perineal hernia: Report of a case with many associated muscular and fascial defects. Ann. Surg. *133*, 255—260 (1951).

Koster, H.: On the supports of the uterus. Amer. J. Obstet. Gynec. *25*, 67—74 (1933).

Kraatz, H. von: Die Haut als Transplantat bei den Ringplastiken zur Behebung der weiblichen Harninkontinenz und zur Fixation eines Scheidenprolaps nach Uterusexstirpation. Zbl. Gynäk. *94*, 299—304 (1972).

Kuhn, R. J. P., Hollyock, V. E.: Observations on the anatomy of the recto-vaginal pouch and septum. Obstet. Gynec. *59*, 445—447 (1982).

Lane, F. E.: Repair of posthysterectomy vaginal vault prolapse. Obstet. Gynec. *20*, 72—77 (1962).

Lahaut, J.: Cure radicale des grands prolapses du rectum. J. Chir. (Paris) *72*, 565—569 (1956).

Langmade, C. F.: Cooper ligament repair of vaginal vault prolapse. Amer. J. Obstet. Gynec. *92*, 601—609 (1965).

Langmade, C. E., Oliver, J. A., White, J. S.: Cooper ligament repair of vaginal vault prolapse twenty-eight years later. Amer. J. Obstet. Gynec. *134*, 16—24 (1978).

Lansman, H. H.: Posthysterectomy vault prolapse: sacral colpopexy with dura mater graft. Obstet. Gynec. *63*, 577—582 (1984).

Lash, A. F., Levin, B.: Roentgenographic diagnosis of vaginal vault hernia. Obstet. Gynec. *20*, 427—433 (1962).

Lawson, J. O. N.: Pelvic anatomy: pelvic floor muscles. Ann. R. Coll. Surg. Engl. *54*, 244—252 (1974).

Lawson, J. O. N.: Motor nerve supply of pelvic floor. Lancet *1*, 999—1000 (1981).

Lee, R. A., Symmonds, R. E.: Surgical repair of posthysterectomy vault prolapse. Amer. J. Obstet. Gynec. *112*, 953—600 (1972).

Le Fort, L. C.: Nouveau procédé pour la guérison du prolapsus utérin. Bull. Gén. Therap. *92*, 337—344 (1877).

Legendre, Bastien: Quoted by Mengert W. F. in Mechanics of uterine support and position. Amer. J. Obstet. Gynec. *31*, 775—782 (1936).

Lin, H.: A new and successful technique of suspending a completely prolapsed vaginal stump. J. Med. Soc. N. J. *75*, 225—227 (1978).

Mackenrodt, A.: Ueber die Ursachen der normalen und pathologischen Lagen des Uterus. Arch. Gynaek. *48*, 393—421 (1895).

Malpas, P.: Genital prolapse and allied conditions. London: Harvey & Blythe 1955.

Marion, G.: De l'obliteration du cul-de-sac de Douglas dans le traitement de certains prolapses uterins. Rev. Gynéc. *13*, 465—470 (1909).

Marshall, C. M.: The newer gynecology: some of its surgical and anatomical implications. Amer. J. Obstet. Gynec. *65*, 773—788 (1953).

Masson, J. C., Simon, H. E.: Vaginal hernia. Surg. Gynec. Obstet. *44*, 36—41 (1927).

Meigs, J. V.: Enterocele or posterior vaginal hernia. Surg. Clin. N. Amer. *27*, 1226—1230 (1947).

Mengert, W. F.: Mechanics of uterine support and position. Amer. J. Obstet. Gynec. *31*, 775—782 (1936).

Miles, L. M.: Pelvic hernia: report of a case of posterior vaginal hernia. Surg. Gynec. Obstet. *42*, 482—490 (1926).

Miller, N. F.: A new method of correcting complete inversion of the vagina. Surg. Gynec. Obstet. *44*, 550—555 (1927).

Moore, H. D.: The results of treatment for complete prolapse of the rectum in the adult patient. Dis. Colon Rectum *20*, 566—569 (1977).

Morgan, C. N.: The surgical anatomy of the ischiorectal space. Proc. R. Soc. Med. *42*, 189—200 (1948).

Moritz, M.: On the nature of the so-called ligaments of Mackenrodt. J. Obstet. Gynaec. Brit. Emp. (Lond.) *23*, 135—138 (1913).

Mortensen, N. J. Mc C., Vellacott, K. D., Wilson, M. G.: Lahaut's operation for rectal prolapse. Ann. R. Coll. Surg. Engl. *66*, 17—18 (1984).

Moschcowitz, A. V.: The pathogenesis, anatomy, and cure of prolapse of the rectum. Surg. Gynec. Obstet. *15*, 7—20 (1912).

McCall, M. L.: Posterior culdeplasty: surgical correction of enterocoele during vaginal hysterectomy; a preliminary report. Obstet. Gynec. *10*, 595—602 (1957).

McLean J. W., Claxton, J. H.: Vaginal prolapse in ewes; part vii: the measurement and effect of intra-abdominal pressure. N. Z. Vet. J. *8*, 51—61 (1960).

Neugebauer, I. A.: Einige Worte über die mediane Vaginalnaht als Mittel zur Beseitigung des Gebärmuttervorfalls. Zbl. Gynäk. *3*, 25—33 (1881).

Nicholls, D. H.: Types of genital prolapse. Postgrad. Med. *46*, 183—187 (1969).

Nicholls, D. H., Milley, P. S.: Surgical significance of the rectovaginal septum. Amer. J. Obstet. Gynec. *108*, 215—220 (1970).

Nicholls, D. H., Milley, P. S., Randall, C. L.: Significance of restoration of normal vaginal depth and axis. Obstet. Gynec. *36*, 251—256 (1970).

Nicholls, D. H.: Types of enterocele and principles underlying choice of operation for repair. Obstet. Gynec. *40*, 257—263 (1972).

Nyulasy, A. J.: The support of the uterus. Surg. Gynec. Obstet. *33*, 53—57 (1921).

Pemberton, J. de, Stalker, L. K.: Surgical treatment of complete rectal prolapse. Ann. Surg. *109*, 799—808 (1939).

Phaneuf, L. E.: Inversion of the vagina and prolapse of the cervix following supracervical hysterectomy and inversion of the vagina following total hysterectomy. Amer. J. Obstet. Gynec. *64*, 739—745 (1952).

Phaneuf, L. E.: Posterior vaginal enterocele. (Hernia of the cul-de-sac of Douglas): a study based on 91 private patients. Obstet. Gynec. *1*, 257—262 (1983).

Popescu, I. et al.: Prolapsul pelvi-perineal dupa histerectomie. Rev. Med. Chir. Soc. Med. Nat. Iasi. *77*, 273—278 (1973).

Porges, R. F., Porges, J. C., Blinick, G.: Mechanisms of uterine support and the pathogenesis of uterine prolapse. Obstet. Gynec. *15*, 711—726 (1960).

Porges, R. F., Porges, J. C.: Theoretical and practical aspects of the surgical correction of pelvic relaxation. Obstet. Gynec. *29*, 450—455 (1967).

Powell, J. L.: Vaginal evisceration following vaginal hysterectomy. Amer. J. Obstet. Gynec. *115*, 276—277 (1973).

Power, R. M. H.: The unstriated muscle fiber of the female pelvis. Amer. J. Obstet. Gynec. *38*, 27—39 (1939).

Power, R. M. H.: Pelvic floor in parturition. Surg. Gynec. Obstet. *83*, 296—311 (1946).

Pratt, J. H.: Secondary operations to correct failures of previous operations for genital prolapse. Clin. Obstet. Gynec. *9*, 1084—1099 (1966).

Puddington, I. E., Guiou, N. M.: Support for posthysterectomy prolapse. Can. Med. Ass. J. *114,* 409 (1976).

Randall, C. L., Nicholls, D. H.: Surgical treatment of vaginal inversion. Obstet. Gynec. *38,* 327—332 (1971).

Ranney, B.: Enterocele, vaginal prolapse, pelvic hernia: recognition and treatment. Amer. J. Obstet. Gynec. *140,* 53—61 (1981).

Ratnam, S. S.: Personal communication. 1981.

Read, C. D.: Enterocele. Amer. J. Obstet. Gynec. *62,* 743—757 (1951).

Richardson, A. C., Williams, G. A.: Treatment of prolapse of the vagina following hysterectomy. Amer. J. Obstet. Gynec. *105,* 90—93 (1969).

Richter, K.: Die chirurgische Anatomie der vaginaefixatio sacrospinalis vaginalis. Ein Beitrag zur operativen Behandlung des Scheidenblindsackprolapses. Geburtsk. u. Frauenheilk. *28,* 321—327 (1968).

Ridley, J. H.: Evaluation of the colpocleisis operation: a report of 58 cases. Amer. J. Obstet. Gynec. *113,* 1114—1119 (1972).

Ridley, J. H.: A composite vaginal vault suspension using fascia lata. Amer. J. Obstet. Gynec. *126,* 590—600 (1976).

Ripstein, C. B., Lanter, B.: Etiology and surgical therapy of massive prolapse of the rectum. Ann. Surg. *157,* 259—264 (1963).

Rust, J. A., Botte, J. M., Howlett, R. J.: Prolapse of the vaginal vault: Improved techniques for the management of the abdominal approach or vaginal approach. Amer. J. Obstet. Gynec. *125,* 768—776 (1976).

Ryan, P.: Observations upon the aetiology and treatment of complete rectal prolapse. Aust. NZ. J. Surg. *50,* 109—115 (1980).

Savage, H.: The surgery, surgical pathology and surgical anatomy of the female pelvic organs. 2nd Ed. London: J. Churchill & Sons 1870.

Scali, P., Blondon, J., Bethoux, A., Gerard, M.: Les operations de soutenement-suspensions par voie haute dans le traitement des prolapsus vaginaux. J. Gynec. Obstet. Biol. Reprod. (Paris) *3,* 365—378 (1974).

Sears, N. P.: The pelvic fascia. Amer. J. Obstet. Gynec. *29,* 834—839 (1935).

Sederl, J.: Zur Operation des Prolapses der blind endigenden Scheide. Geburtsh. u. Frauenheilk. *18,* 824—828 (1958).

Shafik, A.: A new concept of the anatomy of the anal sphincter mechanism and the physiology of defecation. II. Anatomy of the levator ani muscle with special reference to puborectalis. Invest. Urol. *13,* 175—182 (1975).

Shaw, H. N.: Prolapse of the vaginal vault following hysterectomy: a new method of repair. West. J. Surg. Obstet. Gynec. *56,* 127—133 (1948).

Shively, J. P., Chigos, A. D., Bull, A. L.: Surgical correction of enterocele. Trans. Pac. Coast Obstet. Gynec. Soc. *36,* 51—60 (1968).

Sivasuriya, M.: Treatment of vaginal vault prolapse by a modified Gilliam's suspension technique. Singapore Med. J. *15,* 276—270 (1974).

Soichet, S.: Surgical correction of total genital prolapse with retention of sexual function. Obstet. Gynec. *36,* 69—75 (1970).

Steeper, T. A., Rosai, J.: Aggressive angiomyxoma of the female pelvis and perineum. Amer. J. Surg. Pathol. *7*, 463—475 (1983).

Stoddard, F. J., Myers, R. E.: Connective tissue disorders in obstetrics and gynecology. Amer. J. Obstet. Gynec. *102*, 240—243 (1968).

Sturmdorf, A.: Gynoplastic Technology. Philadelphia: F. A. Davis 1919.

Sutton, G. P., Addison, W. A., Livengood, C. H. III, Hammond, C. B.: Life-threatening hemorrhage complicating sacral colpopexy. Amer. J. Obstet. Gynec. *140*, 836—837 (1981).

Sweetser, H. B.: Vaginal hernia. Ann. Surg. *69*, 609—612 (1919).

Symmonds, R. E., Pratt, J. H.: Vaginal prolapse following hysterectomy. Amer. J. Obstet. Gynec. *79*, 899—909 (1960).

Symmonds, R. E.: Personal communication. 1980.

Taylor, R. W.: Pregnancy after pelvic floor repair. Amer. J. Obstet. Gynec. *94*, 35—39 (1966).

Te Linde, R. W.: Enterocele. In: Operative Gynecology. 2nd Ed. Philadelphia: J. B. Lippincott 1953.

Thelander, C. A.: The importance of the uterosacral ligaments in uterine prolapse. Med. J. Aust. *1*, 511—515 (1922).

Thomas, T. G.: Vulvar and vaginal enterocele. N. Y. Med. J. *42*, 705—711 (1885).

Thompson, R.: The myology of the pelvic floor: a contribution to human and comparative anatomy. Newton, Lancs: McCorquodale 1899.

Thurz, A. D.: A method of treating vaginal vault prolapse. J. Obstet. Gynaec. Brit. Comm. *77*, 1041—1042 (1970).

Timonen, S., Nuoranne, E., Meyer, B.: Genital prolapse. Ann. Chir. Gynaec. Fenn. *57*, 363—370 (1968).

Tobin, C. E., Benjamin, J. A.: Anatomical and surgical restudy of Denonvilliers' fascia. Surg. Gynec. Obstet. *80*, 373—388 (1945).

Todd, J. W.: Mesh suspension for vaginal prolapse. Int. Surg. *63*, 91—93 (1978).

Tomlinson, P. A., Alexander, M. S.: Vaginal prolapse after hysterectomy: a surgical problem. Med. J. Aust. *1*, 319 (1974).

Torpin, R.: Prolapsus uteri associated with spina bifida and club feet in newborn infants. Amer. J. Obstet. Gynec. *43*, 892—894 (1942).

Torpin, R.: Excision of the cul-de-sac of Douglas for the surgical cure of hernias through the female caudal wall, including prolapse of the uterus. J. Med. Ass. Ga. *35*, 396—406 (1947).

Turner, S. J.: Complete prolapse of female genital organs: repair with vaginal conservation. Obstet. Gynec. *17*, 69—79 (1961).

Uhlenhuth, E., Wolfe, W. M., Smith, E. M., Middleton, E. B.: The rectovaginal septum. Surg. Gynec. Obstet. *86*, 148—163 (1948).

Ulfelder, H.: The mechanism of pelvic support in women: deductions from a study of the comparative anatomy and physiology of the structures involved. Amer. J. Obstet. Gynec. *72*, 856—864 (1956).

Ulfelder, H.: The normal mechanism of uterine support and its clinical implications. Western J. Surg. Obstet. Gynec. *68*, 81—83 (1960).

Waldeyer-Hartz, W. von: Das Becken topographisch-anatomisch. Mit besonderer Berücksichtigung der Chirurgie und Gynäkologie dargestellt. Bonn: F. Cohen 1899.

Ward, G. G.: Technic of repair of enterocele (posterior vaginal hernia) and rectocele. JAMA *79*, 709—713 (1922).

Ward, G. G.: The operative technique for the repair of rectocele and injury to the pelvic floor. Surg. Gynec. Obstet. *48*, 399—403 (1929).

Ward, G. E.: Ox fascia lata for reconstruction of round ligaments in correcting prolapse of the vagina. Arch. Surg. *36*, 163—170 (1938).

Waters, E. G.: Vaginal prolapse: technic for correction and prevention at hysterectomy. Obstet. Gynec. *8*, 432—436 (1956).

Waters, E. G., Glasser, J. W. H.: Prolapse of the vagina following hysterectomy. Bull. M. Hague Matern. Hosp. *8*, 58—61 (1955).

Weed, J. C., Tyrone, C.: Enterocele: an analysis of 52 cases. Amer. J. Obstet. Gynec. *60*, 324—332 (1950).

Wells, C. S.: Polyvinyl alcohol sponge prosthesis. Proc. R. Soc. Med. *55*, 1083—1084 (1962).

Welsh, F.: Polyethylene sling for procidentia. Br. Med. J. *2*, 280—281 (1967).

Wesson, M. B.: Fasciae of the urogenital triangle. JAMA *81*, 2024—2030 (1923).

Wilensky, A. O., Kaufman, P. A.: Vaginal hernia. Amer. J. Surg. *41*, 31—41 (1940).

Winter, G.: Lehrbuch der gynäkologischen Diagnostik. Unter Mitarbeitung von Carl Ruge. Leipzig: S. Hirzel 1896.

Wyka, Z.: Treatment of complete vaginal prolapse after vaginal surgery. Przegl. Lek. *26*, 509—511 (1970).

Yates, M. J.: An abdominal approach to the repair of posthysterectomy vaginal inversion. Br. J. Obstet. Gynaec. *82*, 817—819 (1975).

Zacharin, R. F.: The suspensory mechanism of the female urethra. J. Anat. *97*, 423—427 (1963).

Zacharin, R. F.: The anatomic supports of the female urethra. Obstet. Gynec. *32*, 754—759 (1968).

Zacharin, R. F.: Genital prolapse in ruminants. Aust. NZ J. Obstet. Gynaec. *9*, 236—239 (1969).

Zacharin, R. F., Hamilton, N. T.: The problem of the large enterocoele. Aust. NZ J. Obstet. Gynaec. *12*, 105—109 (1972).

Zacharin, R. F.: "A Chinese anatomy" — the supporting tissues of the Chinese and Occidental female compared and contrasted. Aust. NZ J. Obstet. Gynaec. *17*, 1—11 (1977).

Zacharin, R. F.: Pulsion enterocoele: review of functional anatomy of the pelvic floor. Obstet. Gynec. *55,* 135—140 (1980).

Zacharin, R. F., Hamilton, N. T.: Pulsion enterocoele: longterm results of an abdominoperineal technique. Obstet. Gynec. *55,* 141—148 (1980).

Zacharin, R. F.: Abdominoperineal urethral suspension in the management of recurrent stress incontinence of urine — a 15 year experience. Obstet. Gynec. *62,* 644—654 (1983).

Zweifel, P.: Vorlesungen über klinische Gynäkologie. Berlin: Hirschwald 1892.

Subject Index